Five Element I

CW01203848

By Taggart King

Published by Pinchbeck Press

www.pinchbeckpress.com
Email: taggart@reiki-evolution.co.uk

Copyright © 2009 Taggart King.

ISBN 978-1-9998852-0-5

Introduction 7

Traditional Chinese Medicine 11

  Basics of TCM 12

  The Basic Components of TCM 14

The Five Elements 21

  Basics of the Five Elements 22

  Five Elements Correspondences 37

  The Correspondences of the Organs 49

  Other Correspondences of the Elements 77

  Five Element Theory: FAQ 85

Experiencing the Five Energies 86

  Five Element Symbols 87

  Five Element Energy Meditations 95

  Feedback from 'Guinea Pigs' 100

Working on Your Self 110

  Monitoring the State of Your Elements 111

  General impressions: an "inner knowing" 114

  Dowsing - General 117

  How to Dowse your Elements 125

  Using Visualisation to Intuit your Elements 131

  Using Physical Movements to Intuit your Elements 141

Five Element Self-Treatments 146

  The simplest Five Element self-treatment...ever! .. 148

Self-treatment through breathing light 151

"Gentle" self-treatments 156

Gentle 'Hands On' Self-Treatment method............. 158

Gentle 'Hands Off' Self-Treatment method............. 166

"Stronger" self-treatments 168

Stronger 'Hands On' Self-Treatment method 172

Stronger 'Hands Off' Self-Treatment method 184

Self-Treatment Case History.................................... 187

Working on Other People 192

Introduction... 193

Perceiving Someone Else's Elements.................... 195

Sensing Over the Hara... 198

Making sense of the imbalances you find............... 203

Some examples... 205

Student Comments About Hara Diagnosis............. 210

Stabilising and Preparing Someone's Elements 213

Treating the Elements.. 214

Introduction... 215

Working on organ pairs.. 215

Treatment Option 1: Treating the Elements Simply 217

Option 2: Treating the Elements using Visualisation
.... 227

Option 3: Treating the Elements using Intent only (and not moving!).. 232

Mixing Five Element Treatments with standard Reiki
.... 238

Treatment Case Histories 240

Subjective differences between Reiki and Five
Element Treatments.. 252

Five Element Treatments: FAQ 254

More Advanced Treatments 256

Narrowing your Focus... 257

The "Organ Focus".. 258

Two New Organs.. 263

"Balanced Presentations".. 264

The "Aspect Focus".. 265

A Worked Example 269

Some Treatment Reports from Students................ 274

Using Organ and Aspect Focus when you Self-treat
.... 280

Treating by 'pushing' some sliders 283

Summary of Treatment Technique............................ 286

Intuiting Imbalances 287

Stabilising the Elements.. 288

Working on Organ Pairs.. 288

Appendix 290

Recommended Reading 290

Dowsing Grid 291

Introduction

Welcome to Five Element Reiki, which as far as I can tell is a unique way of working with Reiki, where you are in effect doing acupuncture without needles, or doing acupressure without pressing on anything, and without having to learn about or focus on the body's meridians or their acupoints.

Five Element Reiki is a way of working with the energies of the five elements of Traditional Chinese Medicine (TCM) so that the meridians and 'organs' associated with each element 'resonate' with the energy you are channelling, removing 'blockages' and bringing a state of balance on all levels.

In this manual you will begin by learning about Traditional Chinese Medicine and the ways that the Five Elements show themselves in our bodies, in our minds and in our emotions.

This is just an overview, but by the end of this section you will know which organs are associated with each element, which emotion, which states of mind and how imbalances might show themselves.

And while this academic knowledge helps us to understand how elemental imbalances show themselves in our body-mind-spirit, and gives us insights into the likely effects of using elemental energies, this knowledge is not essential in order to carry out Five Element Reiki effectively.

You do not need to have a lot of knowledge to be able to use this system safely and effectively, which is nice!

You will then move on to experience the energy of the five elements by carrying out a series of energy meditations using five symbols, you will learn how to detect elemental imbalances within yourself and you will use the five energies to bring your elements into balance.

Next you will learn how to use these energies on other people.

Now, if you are going to balance someone's elements then first you need to know where the imbalances are, so we will be describing methods that you can use to detect energy imbalances in others.

Most of these are based on using your intuition, so I go into a lot of detail and provide many methods and approaches that you can use to access the intuitive knowledge that already resides within you.

In fact, this book almost contains an entire mini-course or masterclass in accessing your intuitive knowledge.

So, once you know where the imbalances are, you can do something about it, so you will learn how to treat someone's elements in order to produce long-term balance.

I present various techniques that you can use to achieve the desired results, in each main section of the manual, so you can experiment and find your own distinctive way with this system, which is very flexible and intuitive.

This manual is comprehensive and detailed. It provides background theory and explains the practical stages in an easy-to-understand way.

You'll find case histories and examples that demonstrate what's possible and the effects that this system can have in people's lives.

Five Element Reiki is simple, it can be practised by anyone who is already at Reiki Second Degree level, and I hope that you find the techniques presented on this course easy to put into practice.

I wish you luck with them.

Taggart King
Reiki Evolution
www.reiki-evolution.co.uk

Traditional
Chinese
Medicine

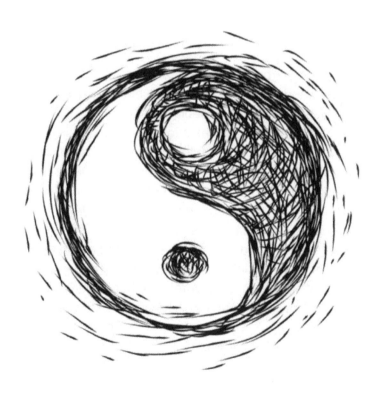

Basics of TCM

What follows is a very general overview of the principles of Traditional Chinese Medicine (TCM) and is designed to show the breadth of its theories, and its application in a wide range of therapies and techniques. For those who would like to investigate this subject in more depth than can be achieved here, we provide a reading list at the end of this manual.

Breadth of TCM

Acupuncture, herbal medicine, massage techniques, diet advice and QiGong are all forms of treatment that are practised in their own special ways. An acupuncturist inserts needles into specific points in various parts of the body, while a herbalist prescribes a variety of herbs, pills, powders and tinctures. QiGong uses movement and exercise to cultivate personal levels of 'chi' and produce balance and health. A Tui Na practitioner uses direct massage techniques. Dietary therapy consists of advice about what to eat which the patient is able to put into practice at home. These disparate areas seem quite unrelated, but there is something that links these outwardly diverse treatments.

The linking thread is the theory of Traditional Chinese Medicine.

History of TCM

TCM has a long history: there is evidence that there was a sophisticated approach to medical problems as long ago as the Shang Dynasty (circa 1,000 BC). Archaeological digs have unearthed early acupuncture needles, and discourses on medical conditions have been discovered inscribed on bones.

Early Asian shamanic practices are believed to be at the foundation of TCM, and the Chinese emphasis on the balancing and governing forces of nature seem to have developed through the observation of the natural world.

By the 1st century AD the first and most important classic text of Chinese Medicine had been completed.

The text was probably compiled over several hundred years and based on the writings of many authors, and takes the form of a dialogue between the legendary 'Yellow Emperor' and his Minister, on the subject of medicine.

The 'Inner Classic' expounds the philosophy of Chinese Medicine and a further section deals with the benefits of acupuncture, herbs, diet and exercise. Over the following centuries, these basic writings were expanded upon, and much of the current practice of TCM reflects traditions that have developed over the last 3,000 years.

Whichever of the above forms of treatment a person chooses to have, the underlying theory comes from the same root, and this root forms the foundation for a unique diagnosis of each individual.

The Basic Components of TCM

There are three main components of the theory of Chinese medicine that are used in diagnosis. Together they enable the practitioner to find the exact energetic cause of a patient's problem.

These are the components:

- Yin and Yang
- The Vital Substances
- The Five Elements

This course concentrates on the five elements and one of the vital substances: Qi.

We will deal with the five elements in detail later, obviously, and here we will just touch on Yin & Yang and the Vital Substances.

Yin and Yang

One of the oldest classics of Chinese Medicine, 'The Yellow Emperor's Classic of Internal Medicine' (referred to above) states that:

> To live in harmony with Yin and Yang means life.
> To live against Yin and Yang means death.
> To live in harmony with Yin and Yang will bring peace.
> To live against Yin and Yang will bring chaos.

These two fundamental forces of the universe are said to be in opposition yet interdependent, to consume each other and to transform into each other.

Nature is seen to group itself into pairs of mutually dependent opposites, for example the concept of 'night' has no meaning without the concept of 'day'; 'up' has no meaning without 'down'.

According to the Chinese view, all things in the universe have Yin and Yang aspects, and though the balance of Yin and Yang will vary, both aspects will always be present.

Each patient has their own particular balance of Yin and Yang, and when people become ill their balance of Yin and Yang will be affected. Sometimes a person will become more Yang in nature; Yang is associated with fire and the fire may start to rage as it is not held in check by the Yin.

On the other hand, sometimes a person may have relatively too much Yin energy which is not held in check by their Yang, and they will experience symptoms of Yang's association with water.

We do not focus on the idea of Yin and Yang on this course.

The Vital Substances

The cells form the basic structure of the human body as far as Western medicine is concerned, and physiology is the Western study of the body's 'normal' functioning. The Vital Substances are their equivalent in Chinese medicine. They describe the main constituents of a person and the functioning of the vital substances could be seen as 'Chinese physiology'.

These are the vital substances:

- Qi
- The Blood
- The Jing Essence
- The Body Fluids
- Shen (mind-spirit)

Qi is familiar to Reiki practitioners! It is called Ki in Japanese. It is the energy that underlies everything in the universe. Condensed it becomes matter, refined it becomes spirit, and everything that is living, moving and vibrating does so because Qi moves through it.

An old Chinese text called the Nan Jing says that "Qi is the root of all human beings". Ted Kaptchuk describes Qi as 'matter on the verge of becoming energy, or energy at the point of materialising'. There are many sorts of Qi: Original Qi, Gathering Qi, Upright Qi, Nutritive Qi, Defensive Qi, Meridian Qi, Liver Qi, Lung Qi and so on and so on.

We do not need to know about these various kinds if Qi on this course.

Blood in Chinese medicine is not the same as the 'blood' that we think of. 'Blood' is described by what it does rather than by what it is, and it is seen as the fluid that nourishes and moisturises the body. It also houses Shen (see later). For example, the symptoms of 'blood deficiency' include:

- frequent pins and needles or cramps due to malnourishment of the muscles and tendons
- dry skin and brittle nails due to lack of moistening of the skin
- constant anxiety, poor memory and lack of concentration due to the blood not 'housing' the Shen

Jing is something that we inherit from our parents and the state of a person's Qi and Blood depend on this 'essence'. The strength of our Jing determines our constitution, it is stored in our kidneys, and it allows us to develop from childhood to adulthood to old age.

The Jing that we inherit at birth is all that we have for the rest of our lives, it varies in amount from one person to another, and most people have an average amount of it. As we get older, our greying hair and failing memories are signs that our Jing is becoming depleted.

Body fluids are referred to as 'Jin Ye' in Chinese medicine. The 'Jin' body fluids are light and watery and are at the exterior of our body. The 'Ye' body fluids are heavier and are found more inside us.

If the body fluids are 'stuck' then the free movement of Qi and Blood in the body can be obstructed. These body fluids are the most 'substantial' of all the vital substances in Chinese medicine!

Shen by contrast is the most 'insubstantial' of all the substances in the body, and it can be said to be a rarefied form of Qi. It could also be said to be our very spirit itself. It is housed in the heart by the Blood.

Shen, Qi and Jing are called 'the Three Treasures', and together they are seen as the basis of our health. The Chinese will often use the term 'Jingshen' as a sort of short-hand term for vitality or vigour, and the term sends us the message that the basis of a healthy life is a good constitution and a strong spirit.

Alongside Yin and Yang and the Vital Substances, knowledge of the five elements and their twelve organs is important in diagnosis so that we can understand any imbalance in an individual.

These latter areas are what this course is all about, and the remainder of this manual deals with these areas in detail, giving their practical relevance to Reiki practitioners.

The Five Elements

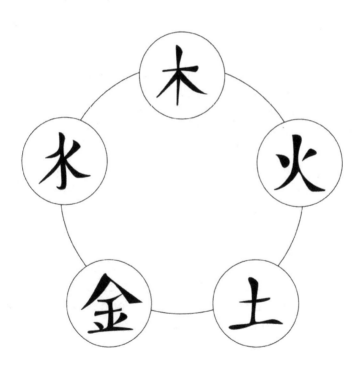

Basics of the Five Elements

The phrase 'five elements' seem to me to be a bit of a misnomer, because it suggests to me something fixed and solid. But the elements are creative processes, they are forces, they are phases, functions and movements; they are dynamic, interact with each other in an endless dance, and manifest or condense in different aspects of our body-mind-spirit. The Five Elements are different characteristics of nature imprinted on all levels of our body-mind-spirit. In fact, the philosophical origins of Chinese medicine have grown out of the tenets of Taoism, which bases much of its thinking on the observation of the natural world.

Each 'element' is a badge that represents a range of related functions and qualities. For example, Wood represents active functions that are in a growing phase, Fire represents functions that have reached a maximal state of activity. Metal represents functions that are in a state of decline, whereas Water represents functions that have reached a maximal state of rest and are about to change their direction of activity. Earth represents balance and neutrality, and can be seen as a 'buffer' between the other phases.

So if we translate these principles into the seasons of the year, then Wood represents the growth of spring, Fire represents the high activity of summer, Metal represents the decline of autumn and Water represents the quiet waiting period of winter. Earth is seen as representing the transition between each season, or can be seen as 'Indian Summer', the pause that nature takes between the activity of summer (Fire) and the decline of autumn (Metal).

Over time, a wider and wider range of correspondences has developed: everything from colours, sounds, odours and taste sensations, to emotions, animals, grains, plants, planets and even dynasties. The connections between the elements and the anatomical organs, with the emotions and mental/spiritual states, are the areas that we are most concerned with in this course. Some of the connections have come through the application of, for example, the idea of wooden-ness (the dynamic phase) to the physical body, and some have come through observation. So the emotion anger is associated with Wood, not because anger is inherently 'wooden' in nature, but because careful observation of people has shown that disturbances in anger are associated with the Liver, an 'organ' of Wood.

Ultimately, everything in the universe is Wood, Fire, Earth, Metal or Water.

The Five Phases theory was first set down in a coherent way by Zou Yen (350 BCE - 270 BCE approx.), whereas

Yin-Yang theory stretches back into China's distant, distant past. The Five Virtues or Five Powers were used at that time to arrive at the proper colours, musical notes and instruments, or sacrifices, that were appropriate to different dynasties or emperors, and only later became an important part of Chinese medical thought. The Yin-Yang and Five Phase theories were uncomfortable bedfellows for a long time, and it was only in the Han Dynasty - which was a time of great eclecticism and synthesis - that the two systems started to come together in Chinese medicine. The Five Elements are a working proposition to explain the interconnectedness of all aspects of our body-mind-spirit, rather than rigid dogma that should be applied in all circumstances.

Interconnectedness

The five elements do not stand alone. They are linked together in an endless cycle, a fascinating and complicated interplay. What happens to one element can have knock-on effects on the others. In the diagram below you can see the elements arranged around the edges of a circle, and explanations that describe two ways in which the elements interact.

The Nourishment Cycle

Moving clockwise round the circle, the elements give support and nourishment to each other, rather like a parent giving support and nourishment to an offspring.

So Fire supports Earth, Earth supports Metal, Metal supports Water, Water supports Wood, and Wood supports Fire. In terms of the natural world, you can imagine that wood burns to produce fire, fire when it has burnt produces ashes which are earth, deep down in earth metals can be found, water condenses on metal surfaces, and water nourishes the growth of wood. These connections are rooted in the observation of the natural world.

When wood is weak or depleted, fire may become depleted also. The emotion of wood is anger, and the emotion of fire is joy, so someone who has wood depletion, and cannot express anger - or suppresses anger - may not be able to fully express joy either. In the Chinese view of things, the full expression of joy would be accompanied by the full expression of anger.

Diagram of the Nourishment Cycle

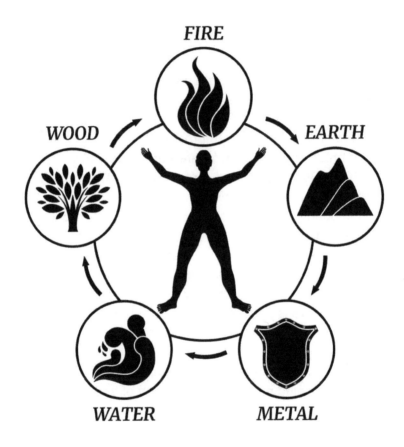

The Control Cycle

There is another way that the elements are connected to each other, and you can see this on the diagram overleaf too. Each element controls another element, rather like a grandparent giving guidance and advice to a grandchild. In more traditional societies, the parents would be engaged in working to support the family, while the grandparents' role was to guide and bring up the children of the extended household.

You can see from the diagram that Fire controls Metal (fire can melt metal), Earth controls Water (earth can dam a river), Metal controls Wood (an axe can fell a tree), Water controls Fire (water can extinguish a fire) and Wood controls Earth (wood can be used to fence off and control an area of land). These connections are again rooted in the observation of the natural world.

So if Water is too strong, Fire may become depleted. On the other hand, if Water is too weak, Fire may burn uncontrolled.

Diagram of the Nourishment and Control Cycles

The Nourishment Cycle moves clockwise round the circle

The Control Cycle follows the straight lines: one element controls the other

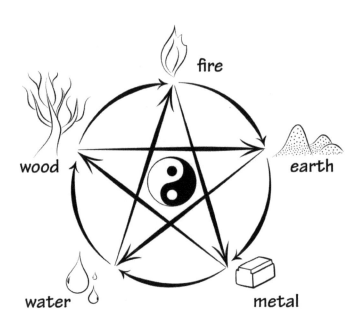

The Complexity of TCM

These descriptions give a hint of the complexity of TCM. If one has a lung problem, most likely there may be a problem with Metal, and that is the root cause.

However, the root cause may be elsewhere:

Metal may be affected because of an imbalance in its supporting element (Earth) or because of an imbalance in its controlling element (Fire). TCM searches for the root cause, and so there would be many different sorts of treatments for what would seem to be the same medical condition.

In fact, what is described above is not the end of the story, because there are two other ways in which the elements can interconnect.

If an element is severely depleted, and needs more energy than is contained within it, then it may start to drain energy from the element that supports it.

So a long-term medical problem related to Earth may start to drain, and have a knock-on effect on, Fire, the element that supports it.

There is also a relationship described as a rebellious grandchild, where too much Chi in one element can start to deplete the element that is trying to control it.

The Simplicity of Five Element Reiki

The above demonstrates that there is a great deal of depth in TCM; this is an understatement!

Fortunately, success with Five Element Reiki does not depend on such detail. It does not depend on tricky diagnostic procedures such as the taking of the six pulses, for example, which is done by acupuncturists to find exactly which meridian is out of balance, and to determine the precise root cause of a condition.

With Five Element Reiki we are bringing all the elements into balance by using their characteristic energies, and we are flushing through affected elements and their associated 'organs' to produce balance on all levels, spending more time on the elements that are most out of balance.

For us, the precise root cause does not need to be determined: we will be balancing it, and it's knock-on effects, at the same time.

The Meridian System and 'Organs'

Meridians are channels of energy running throughout our bodies, and each meridian is related to a particular body 'organ' from which it takes its name. There are twelve major meridians and number of minor meridians related to each organ, and you will have seen diagrams or posters depicting the course of the various meridians over the surface of the human body. Although the majority of the meridians are related to physical organs that we in the West would recognise, not all of them are, and they do not necessarily work on the same physical basis.

For example, there are two 'organs' that are unknown to Western physiology: the Pericardium (or Heart Protector) and the Triple Burner, Sanjiao, or Triple Heater. The Pericardium protects the heart from emotional upsets and 'knocks', and protects us from external 'attacks' such as infections. The Triple Heater harmonises the organs and ensures the safe passage of energy and fluids through our bodies; malfunctioning is seen as causing Chi or body fluids to become blocked in our systems.

The word 'organ' does not have the same meaning in Chinese medicine as we would understand in the West when we think of the liver or the heart, for example. Each organ also has a much wider range of associations, characteristics, functions and influence than the physical organs we perceive in the West, and we are going to look at this in more detail later on. Each 'organ' functions on all levels of our body-mind-spirit, part of an overall dynamic energy process.

On this course the meridians and particularly the 'organs' are important because each organ is allocated to a particular element, so if we want to work on Wood then we can focus energy on the 'organs' of Wood: Liver and Gall Bladder, and their associated meridians. We will we be focusing energy on these organs and we will be sending the organ's characteristic energy through it, intensifying the beneficial effect by making the 'organ' and its meridian resonate at its characteristic frequency. When we work on the Liver and the Gall Bladder we will be sending Wood energy through those organs, to produce balance in Wood on a deep level. We will produce balance in all the various ramifications and associations of Wood: anger, planning, decision-making, the tendons, the eyes, tears, and so on (see later discussions of the associations of each element).

Usually two organs represent each element, one Yin organ and one Yang organ, one solid organ and one hollow organ, and listed below are the major meridians/organs and their associated element. You can also see them depicted in the diagram on the next page:

| **Wood** | Liver |
| | Gall Bladder |

Fire	Heart
	Small Intestine
	(Heart protector)
	(Triple Heater)

| **Earth** | Spleen/Pancreas |
| | Stomach |

| **Metal** | Lung |
| | Large Intestine |

| **Water** | Kidney |
| | Bladder |

The Yin organs are the solid organs: Liver, Heart, Heart Protector, Spleen/Pancreas, Lung and Kidney. These organs are considered to be deeper in the body and are concerned with the manufacture, storage and regulation of the fundamental substances. They each have an emotion associated with them.

The Yang organs are hollow: Gall Bladder, Small Intestine, Triple Heater, Stomach, Large Intestine and Bladder. These organs are considered to be closer to the surface of the body, and have the functions of receiving, separating, distributing and excreting body substances.

Interestingly, in the same way that one element supports another in a continuous cycle, in TCM one organ/meridian can be seen as supporting the next. So the Heart supports and nourishes the Spleen, and this in turn nourishes the Lungs. The Lungs support the Kidneys, and these nourish the Liver. The Liver supports the Heart and so on.

There are two other meridians outside the element classification, and they run down the front and back of the body in the midline. These meridians will be familiar to those carrying out the microcosmic orbit meditation: The Conception and Governing Vessels.

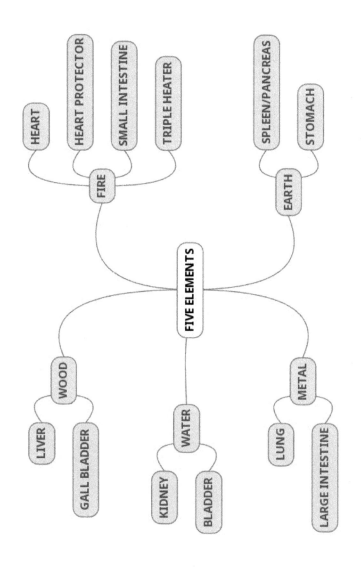

35

Five Elements Correspondences

In this section I want to touch on some of the important correspondences of the elements, for example the emotions, the 'organs', meridians and the various body parts connected with each element.

The usefulness of this is that if you know that Metal is reflected in the emotion of grief, represents the lungs and the large intestine, and also the skin, then you can understand that:

- Constipation may be connected with suppressed grief
- Helping someone to release suppressed grief can lead to skin condition improving, as happened a while ago with someone I was working on

There are many, many correspondences to each element, and some are not so relevant for our purposes. Please see the reading list if you wish to learn more.

The Emotions of the Elements

In Traditional Chinese medicine there are a number of internal causes of disharmony that are termed the 'seven emotions'. They are Anger, Joy, Sadness, Grief, Pensiveness, Fear and Fright. Sadness and Grief, and Fear and Fright, may be taken together, giving five basic causes of disharmony, one for each element.

In traditional Chinese medicine the emphasis is on balance, so none of the seven emotions are considered to be 'good' or 'bad' in themselves. What is important is how they balance. Negative connotations are not placed on anger, or any of the other emotions of the elements, though Western society tends to frown on the expression of anger and so this emotion tends to become suppressed, with knock-on effects in other areas (see later). All the emotions have their place in a healthy individual and they should be felt and expressed. Most people experience a wide range of emotions that vary in intensity; some are appropriate and adaptive, others are less so. Too much Joy is as out of balance as too much Grief, but the disharmony will express itself in a different way.

In this section I touch on the emotional associations of each element, and then we will move on to look at more basic characteristics of each element, particularly their associated 'organs', and the ramifications of these on various levels.

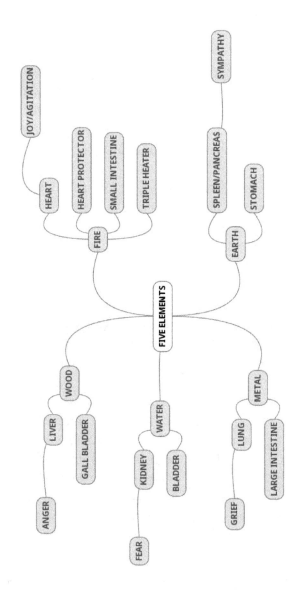

FIVE ELEMENTS

FIRE
- HEART — JOY/AGITATION
- HEART PROTECTOR
- SMALL INTESTINE
- TRIPLE HEATER

EARTH
- SPLEEN/PANCREAS — SYMPATHY
- STOMACH

WOOD
- LIVER — ANGER
- GALL BLADDER

WATER
- KIDNEY — FEAR
- BLADDER

METAL
- LUNG — GRIEF
- LARGE INTESTINE

Wood: Anger

The emotion of Wood is anger and aggression, together with the associated feelings of irritability, hatred, fury and rage, resentment and frustration. Anger and aggression are a sign of an obstacle in our path, preventing us from growing, and we become frustrated if we cannot find the space for expression.

Creativity is an element of wood and so when people find themselves stuck creatively, anger and aggression can become a problem. Also creativity is a useful tool for expression and can be considered as a means to help someone maintain more balance in Wood.

Anger and aggression are seen as positive emotions that allow us to overcome impediments to our growth, but irritability, hatred, rage and fury are seen as signs of a Wood imbalance, and are not healthy emotions.

Rage, for example, can be seen as anger that has lost its purpose and gone out of control. We speak of 'blind rage'. A person might be continually angry with themselves or on edge with others, irritable and always wanting to pick a fight with someone. They might feel 'stuck', paralysed because they are unable to escape their fury. Annoyance and irritability can also be seen as energies that have yet to be focused.

If a person keeps their rage inside, it can seethe under a cold and polite surface; underneath there may be a feeling of great frustration or inner conflict, and if the rage ever broke free there might be dangerous consequences. Such suppressed aggression also goes hand in hand with suppressed and inhibited sexuality, so healthy sexual behaviour is seen as related to healthy aggressive behaviour.

Emotional imbalances in Wood can be expressed in different ways. For example, chronic irritability and unreasonable temper tantrums can be indicative of an excess of chi in the Gall Bladder. This can cause headaches in the crown and at the temples, and if this state of rage continues not to be expressed or cleared out then high blood pressure or Gallstones might result.

A person may exhibit suppressed rage: sarcasm, cynicism, bitterness and a general inability to become angry. This can be associated with apathy, sluggishness, resignation and depression, which in themselves are what we might see in a person who has given up making plans and manifesting goals (some of the other characteristics of the Liver and the Gall Bladder - see later).

Such an outlook may have arisen because a person has been confronted continually with obstacles to their self-realisation. Continued failure can lead people to give up, perhaps leading to alcoholism or drug addiction, which are in themselves injurious to the Liver.

41

The last two paragraphs represent an excess of Yang energy in Wood, and a deficiency of Yang energy in Wood respectively. A lack of Yang energy might be caused by too much Yin energy in the Liver (the Yin organ) or a lack of Yang energy in the Gall Bladder (the Yang organ). This is where it all gets rather complicated, and for the purposes of this course, fortunately, we do not need to go deeper into the Yin and Yang characteristics of the elements, the organs and their emotions!

If over the years a person cannot express and clear their hatred and rage, and turn these emotions into a positive striving towards goals, then the aggression can turn itself against the person's own body, leading to gout, arthritis, rheumatism, and other auto-immune or auto-aggressive disorders. Interestingly, these diseases are more often found in women, and in patriarchal cultures women have less opportunity than men do to express themselves, especially when it comes to carrying through with an idea or venting their anger.

The healthy situation is where anger and aggression can be expressed and then will turn naturally into joy and love, the emotions associated with Fire, the element which follows Wood in the endless cycle of the elements.

Fire: Joy

In Chinese medicine the concept of Joy refers more to a state of agitation or over-excitement rather than our more passive notion of deep contentment, and Joy is related to the Heart.

An imbalance in Fire will show itself as a lack of joy, or joy in excess, and both are harmful. If someone has an insatiable desire for permanent joy, and this is pursued relentlessly through work or play, then this can put too much stress on Fire and lead to, for example, palpitations and high blood pressure.

Fire also governs the blood vessels. Excessive striving for joy is not healthy, and the stress involved may include a great deal of sexual frustration.

An imbalance in fire almost always revolves around a relationship in the person's life, according to one author.

Since the elements are connected, and Wood supports Fire, a lack of chi in Wood - leading to suppression of anger - can also lead to a suppression in joy, so a person who is unable to properly express anger may be unable to fully experience joy.

Earth: Sympathy

Earth expresses itself through compassion, recognition, sympathy and a feeling of love and unity with one's environment, through a basic feeling that one is welcome and at home where one is at that moment. There is a self-assurance that does not need to be proven, an inner security and calmness.

So people with a deficiency in Earth feel insecure, sometimes begging for attention and affection. Beneath this behaviour lies the belief that warmth and affection could be taken away or denied. Childhood experiences can lead to this belief becoming established in a person. In fact, the search for missing security is the driving force and main occupation of people with a 'weak' Earth. They look for this security in eating or smoking, they might be overly affectionate - grasping for love - and constantly looking for the security of motherly love in their relationships. They can hide their fear of abandonment behind a romantic ideal of love and partnership.

The basic emotion of Earth is sympathy or compassion, so an imbalance in Earth can show itself in a person who lacks compassion, or who does not seem to enter into relationships with others. The affairs of others do not seem to touch them very much, and a critical stance towards others can go hand in hand with this, with harsh judgements and low tolerance masking an underlying insecurity. Voicing criticisms helps to build up the person's sense of superiority.

An imbalance could show itself as self-pity and constant whining about one's own problems, in martyrdom. An example that I read was that of a woman who sacrifices herself for her husband and children, not treating herself to anything; she can moan and point to her destiny as the reason for this. Maybe the person would seek sympathy continually, obsessively, and perhaps even make up symptoms to attract more compassion towards them. By contrast, they might be unable to receive sympathy themselves. Whether someone asks for sympathy all the time, or cannot receive it, they are 'stuck' and aren't able to move easily in and out of the emotion. In a balanced person, the emotions can flow freely.

So a person with a healthy Earth has an 'inner abundance' from which to give and care for others, rather like the fullness and abundance that nature displays in late summer. When this element is deficient, this 'sweetness' can turn into a constant overflow of 'sticky' emotional outbursts, or over-exaggerated generosity which serves to make others dependent; think of a mother who prevents her children from becoming adults by limiting their responsibilities and not allowing them to make decisions. Perhaps the person would be far too sympathetic, to the point of being obsequious.

Metal: Grief

If we follow the analogy of the seasons, and remember Metal's association with autumn, then we can imagine the state of mind in simple agricultural communities: wondering how they are going to last the winter as the cold dark days approach. There would be worries about the future, and Metal imbalance can display itself in just such a worry, but in an exaggerated form, with perhaps a pessimistic attitude, a hopelessness. By contrast, a healthy Metal would display trust in life, optimism and a positive view of the future.

The feeling autumn is sadness, a sadness that fills us when we have to leave something that has be come precious and dear to us. This feeling is exaggerated in people who are unable to let go of something that they can never get back. Thus the emotion of Metal is grief. An imbalance in Metal will show itself as being unable to grieve, suppressing grief, or in feeling a sense of loss continually, perhaps a sadness about things that have not yet happened, when we realise that we have not taken advantage of our opportunities. Grief is a natural and a healthy process, of course, but a person who is overwhelmed by sorrow is likely to be displaying a Metal imbalance. Someone who is going through grief may experience breathing difficulties or bowel problems for a while, and sometimes these problems may persist; we will see later that the Lungs and the Large Intestine are the 'organs' of Metal.

Our Lungs hold the emotion of Grief, and they are directly involved in the expression of this emotion: a normal and healthy expression of grief and sadness is sobbing that originates in the depths of our lungs, deep breaths and the expulsion of air with the sob. Sadness that remains and becomes chronic can create a disharmony in the Lungs, weakening Lung chi, and this will interfere with the Lungs' many functions and energetic processes.

Water: Fear

The emotion of Water is fear, which is a healthy and natural response to dangerous situations, a normal and adaptive human emotion. We fear something concrete, recognise the danger in time, and we take action to get away from something that is threatening to us. Fear ensures our survival.

But anxiety and terror are more intense because they are emotional states where the threat can't be assessed properly, and in fact the threat may be imaginary. Anxiety exists when a threat can't be judged correctly, or may no longer exist.

We develop anxiety when we isolate ourselves and we aren't in harmony with things and people around us any more. Being able to 'resonate' with our environment is a characteristic of Water: to be soft, to surrender oneself and to not offer any resistance.

So a serious imbalance in Water can show itself as panic attacks, paranoia, a persecution complex, fear of the dark, a variety of phobias or even a general amorphous feeling of dread or foreboding, a pervading sense of anxiety about life. We may become rigid, immovable and paralysed by fear.

Fear involves holding on to an anxiety rather than letting it go and, rather like a river that has been dammed; one can feel overwhelmed, inundated, sinking into despair. Only when the anxiety has been released can we move forward.

The Correspondences of the Organs

Each element is represented by a couple of 'organs', and in the case of Fire, by four 'organs' - two of which do not have Western anatomical counterparts.

The 'organs' for TCM purposes are much, much more than what we think of in the West.

Each organ has a number of correspondences attached to it, so when in TCM someone thinks of the Liver, they are not just imagining the anatomical structure, but also anger - as we have seen above - and the ability to plan ahead.

The 'organs' operate on all levels of the body-mind-spirit, they are energy fields that resonate throughout our being and exhibit their characteristics in different ways.

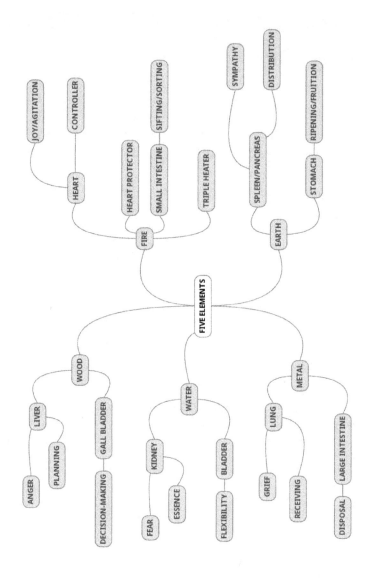

50

Wood: Planning and Decision-Making

Wood brings forth the desire for movement and growth. Its nature is expansion, growing in all directions. It brings forth the creative processes of planning and decision-making. It gives us the desire to undertake a new project, to set sail for new horizons and new discoveries. Wood is represented by the Liver (yin organ) and the Gall Bladder (yang organ).

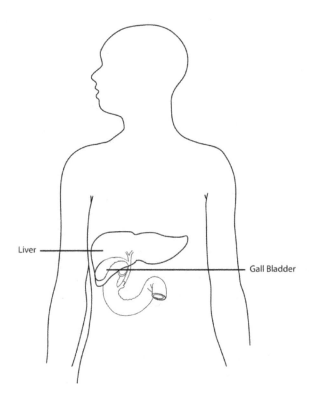

Liver

Gall Bladder

The Liver represents the ability to make plans and to see life on a material level; it embodies the power of imagination and creative energy that results in growth.

It is the inventor, the discoverer. It sees the meaning of life. It develops the vision, the plan. Every new idea that we take hold of, every new concept, broadens our horizons. We take risks and go into the unknown.

We grow, and growth or expansion is the essence of Wood.

You might imagine that when this ability falters then some symptom would arise. For example, a migraine may appear when Liver energy is out of balance, and you could see this as frustration with the system because plans were not made or followed.

So a person with a Wood imbalance might say that they felt 'jammed up in the head so that I can't think, or plan, or do anything'.

Related to the Liver's planning is the Gall Bladder's function in decision making: the ability to assert our needs in the outer world.

If you see the Liver as an architect, then the Gall Bladder is the builder who makes the decisions and arrangements necessary for the blueprints to become a reality. Imagine a person who has difficulty in making decisions, even very little simple ones, and you are thinking of someone with a Gall Bladder imbalance.

The two functions of Liver and Gall Bladder are very closely connected. Without an all-encompassing concept, the decisions in day-to-day life are incoherent, and similarly the best plans and projects are worthless if they cannot be carried out.

Depression and resignation may have their roots in a Wood disorder: the vision is missing, the plan is lacking, or a person may have many plans and ideas but cannot make them into reality.

Fire: Controlling, Sifting, Protecting and Warming

Fire is the only element that is represented by four organs: the Heart (yin organ) and Small Intestine (yang organ), the Heart Protector (yin organ) and the Triple Heater (yang organ). The Heart Protector is also known as the Pericardium or the Circulation Sex and, along with the Triple Heater or Sanjiao, has no physical Western counterpart.

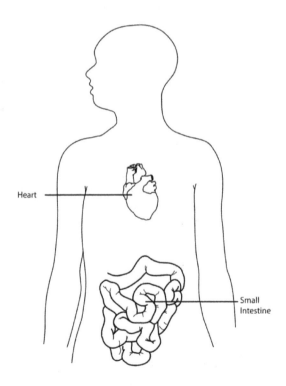

Heart

Small Intestine

The movement of Fire is vertically upward, from deep in the earth up into the sky, from the material to the spiritual, from unawareness to consciousness.

On the mental-emotional level, Fire brings out joy, dancing, laughter, awareness, and the ability to have an encompassing view of things.

The Heart can be viewed as a 'supreme controller' overseeing the workings of the body-mind-spirit, and in Japanese acupuncture writings the Heart is seen as so sacred that it is not treated directly.

An imbalance in Heart energy is like chaos ruling in a kingdom, with a lack of peace and harmony, and leads to feeling a kind of inner panic and loss of control. The Heart is seen as the centre of consciousness, feelings and thoughts, and is one of the places where 'Shen' resides.

Shen can be translated as spirit or soul. A person is said to 'have spirit' and this gives an idea of what is intended by the word Shen.

Shen lives in the heart, its Lower House, and here it makes sure we have balanced feelings and a clear, honest way of speaking. Its higher house is the third eye chakra, where it brings forth clarity of thought and a conscious life direction.

When a person has these characteristics, then their Shen is powerful and healthy, and it is said that you can se this by a sparkle or light in the eyes.

If Shen is confused or lacking in energy then it is noticeable in unclear thinking or an inability to organise thoughts, in speech defects like lisping, stammering, stuttering or even muteness.

It produces emotions full of highs and lows: one minute you are shouting for joy and the next you want to die. This description would fit with hysteria and manic depression also. A dispersed and confused Shen shows itself in nervousness, fearfulness, stage fright, insomnia and dull, unfocused eyes, all caused by a disturbance in Fire.

If there is too much energy in the Heart then there can be talkativeness, excessive perspiration and nervous tension. People believe that they must do everything themselves and not delegate, they must keep control of everything and they are incapable of letting other people take responsibility.

This behaviour equates with the 'Type A' personality - manager sickness - with its stress-related illnesses from high blood pressure to heart attacks. This imbalance is usually connected with an energy deficiency in Water, the element that controls Fire.

On the other hand, when the energy in the Heart is weak, a person may become unable to express themselves clearly, or it may result in partial or total muteness, and a dulled or non-functional sense of taste in both the gastronomical sense and in terms of the psyche.

The Heart Protector, or Pericardium, is seen as a 'buffer' that takes the bumps and bruises that would otherwise go straight to the heart and disturb the integrity of the body-mind, so the Heart Protector allows the 'supreme controller' to carry on its work without interruption. It works as a bodyguard.

On an emotional level, the Heart Protector helps to protect the 'emotional' heart, and it brings out the ability to be generous to oneself and to others, to radiate warmth and to love. It also affords us the ability to give and the ability to accept complaints, criticism and love from others.

A healthy Pericardium produces a person who is able to speak from the heart and be cordial and affectionate, enthusiastic, humorous and 'hearty'. The opposite of this can be seen in someone who is 'cold-hearted' or small-minded, someone who has a 'heart of stone'.

On a physical level, the Pericardium meridian would be treated when there were problems like heart pains, angina, tachycardia, heartbeat irregularities or circulatory problems. The Heart Protector governs the 'pulse of life'.

The Small Intestine can be seen as separating the pure from the impure, sorting and grading and redistributing, and this is seen as happening on all levels.

The Small Intestine sorts particles of food: keeping those with nutritional value and passing on the rest as waste, but you can also see this process carrying on at the emotional level, and at the mental level, with the sorting and sifting, the assimilation, of ideas and thoughts.

An energy deficit in the Small Intestine is displayed in a person who takes in knowledge, convictions and beliefs from others in an 'undigested' form, and they are unable to develop personal views and belief systems out of this. It is said that the appearance of a person who is able to assimilate is displayed through a fine, silent laughing in the eyes and around the lips.

If this organ is out of balance, then we may see symptoms that express confusion of the body-mind. For example, hearing difficulties could be seen as an inability to sort sounds effectively, and digestive problems could be seen in a similar light.

None of the elements exist in isolation, separate and unaffected by the others, so if there is an absence of proper sorting, if there is unclear information coming through, then decision-making is going to be affected (the realm of the Gall Bladder).

The functions of the Triple Heater are closely connected with those of the Heart Protector; in fact it is 'assigned' to the Pericardium. Again it does not have a Western physical counterpart, and its functions are protective. It is the most complex of the 'organs'.

The Triple Heater's function is to guard all the body's organs and control their temperature. The torso is seen as being split into three 'burning spaces' or 'burning cavities', with each space corresponding to certain organs.

The upper space contains the Heart and Lungs, the middle space contains the Stomach, Spleen, Gall Bladder, Liver and Small Intestine, and the lower space contains the Large Intestine, Bladder and Kidneys.

Thus the upper space is concerned with respiration, the middle with digestion, and the lower with elimination and reproduction. The Triple Heater co-ordinates these three areas of the body.

For example, it co-ordinates the depth and frequency of the breath in relation to digestion and sexuality, it maintains the body's temperature at optimum levels within the three burning spaces, so that the organs can carry out their functions in harmony.

Because the Triple Heater is so complex it is the easiest to bring out of balance, and in Acupuncture the Triple Heater would be considered whenever there was an imbalance in the energy of one of the organs, otherwise the cause of an illness might be misdiagnosed.

In Five Element Reiki we are not working on the level of dealing with energy imbalances in a particular organ, but we focus on bringing balance to each element in its entirety. By balancing an element and flushing its energy through its organs, we are bringing its organs into balance, and bringing balance to the other correspondences of that element. By balancing Fire, and flushing Fire Energy through its organs, we will be bringing the Triple Heater into balance without having to consider it specifically, though we will focus energy on it, and the Heart Protector, using intent.

Finally, what does balanced Fire bring to us? Well, when the Fire element is balanced in a person, summer brings us joy and fulfilment. We have an inner balance from which to oversee events, we know when to speak and we know when to remain silent. We can feel joy without becoming excessive. We can steer and lead others, while knowing when the time is right to pull back. Our eyes glow, we know goodness and magnanimity, and we have good taste.

Earth: Distribution and Ripening

Earth represents the time of year of harvesting, sorting, collecting together and storing. While spring looks forward, and summer enjoys the pleasures of the present, late summer - Earth - looks back at what was, and processes it. Earth is the pause between the upward and outward movements of Wood and Fire, and the inward and downward movements of Metal and Water that follow it.

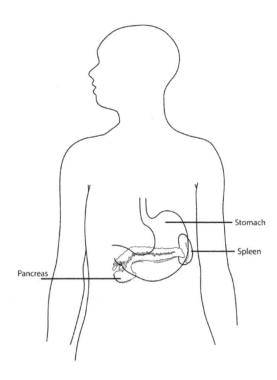

Stomach

Spleen

Pancreas

Earth is also the transition between each season or phase, the time for looking inside and collecting oneself; Earth's direction is horizontal, a closed circle.

On a mental level, Earth can be described in terms of the late summer: gathering, processing, selecting, mental nourishment, survival, and gaining the wisdom that gives us the security to deal with difficult situations in life.

The Spleen-Pancreas holds qualities like logical thinking, a rational intellect, the ability be critical, the ability to think things over, and a good memory. The downside of the Spleen-Pancreas is represented by worrying about a thousand and one things, brooding over the past, and indulging in reminiscences.

An 'over-stimulated' Spleen can show itself in greed for knowledge and the latest news, and an addiction to reading. The most characteristic example of this is the person who accumulates knowledge about detailed areas of human life.

This is the type of knowledge that specialists have: concentrated without seeing the context, the connection to the bigger picture. Another characteristic of an excess energy in the Spleen is seen in the person who can't stop thinking, who has to think through and consider everything.

Yet another example would be the one-sided advocates of science and reason, people who judge and reject every other way of looking at things.

These people are said to compensate for a deficit in Earth by mentally clinging to an apparent security in the logical verification of things. Compulsive behaviour, fixed ideas, obsessions and a passion for collecting that has become obsessive, also represent an excess of energy in the Spleen.

It is interesting at this point to note that it is not only desirable to have balance between the elements, but to also have balance within an element. The energy in earth has to express itself on many levels: physical, mental, emotional etc.

If a person takes up a huge amount of energy in digestion and nourishment then there will not be a great deal of energy left over for thought and reflection. If lots of Earth energy is used up in intellectual activity, then there will be a deficit on the emotional level, leading to a lack of compassion.

Excessive intellectual activity can also produce problems on the physical level, with allergies, menstrual problems, stomach ulcers or metabolic disorders.

The Spleen and the Stomach are good examples of the way that Chinese medicine interprets the idea of an 'organ' differently from Western medicine, even on an organic level. The 'Spleen' for example is seen as encompassing the part of the Pancreas that produces digestive enzymes used in the Duodenum.

The 'Stomach' is seen as including the duodenum and the first six inches of the Small Intestine, which is why digestion, nourishment, assimilation and absorption are classified under the heading of 'Earth'.

The 'Spleen' also represents the lymphatic system: nodes, vessels, tonsils and thymus, it represents the red bone marrow and the mucous membrane of the intestines, since they have a large lymphatic component.

So the idea of 'nourishment' also extends to providing oxygen - via the red blood cells - to every cell in the body.

So the 'Spleen' oversees the transportation of water from the tissues back into the bloodstream, the absorption of fat from the intestine into the lymph system, the production of white blood cells and the storage and breakdown of red blood cells.

The Spleen is the 'mother organ' of the whole body. It regulates the distribution of water and blood, it nourishes the body, and it maintains the integrity of the body through the immune system.

It is also seen as responsible for fertility, pregnancy and birth, together with the Kidney and the Uterus (an extraordinary organ that is not assigned to an element). The breasts are assigned to Earth.

The Spleen is important, and can be seen as being responsible for distribution, and the transport of energy throughout the body-mind. If there is a Spleen-Pancreas imbalance then other parts of the body-mind wouldn't get the energy they need, and for this reason it is said that the 'five viscera' all get their breath of life from the 'Spleen'.

The Stomach can be seen as the organ that receives nourishment, integrates it and brings it to fruition, and then passes on the food energy to be distributed by the Spleen. The Stomach is almost the most important function in the body-mind because our energy feeds from it, and it takes in every aspect of our lives.

If there is a Stomach imbalance then we cannot get the proper benefit from what we take in, whether this is food for our body or food for our mind. What we take in won't be utilised properly.

If we can't get energy from our food properly then we will feel weak, lethargic, we will be depleted and debilitated. Obviously, many digestive problems are associated with an Earth imbalance.

So in practice, Earth imbalances could show as various disorders of the digestive system like indigestion, gastritis, gastric or duodenal ulcers, incomplete digestion, pancreatitis, diarrhoea and constipation.

The immune system could display allergies, auto-immune diseases, immune deficiencies, a tendency towards illness, menstrual problems, infertility, pain and swelling in the breasts, inflammation of the mammary glands, problems with lactating, skin diseases, oedema, as well as diseases of the lymph nodes and lymphatic vessels.

On a different note, disturbances in the natural rhythm of life point to an Earth imbalance. The rhythms of sleeping and waking, of appetite and digestion, breathing, the menstrual cycle would all depend on a balanced Earth. In early Chinese writings on the five elements, Earth was in the centre, and Wood, Fire, Metal and Water were arranged around it.

Not only that, but there were medical and spiritual schools based on handling every physical and spiritual complaint by bringing Earth into balance in a variety of ways encompassing the use of herbs, massage, acupuncture focusing on the Spleen and Stomach meridians, and mental and physical exercises.

Metal: Receiving and Waste Disposal

Metal, the element of autumn, represents concentration, condensation, drawing in; Metal is concentrated energy, the opposite of Wood. Metal is represented by the Lungs and the Large Intestine, the 'organs' responsible for energy transfer on all levels; they receive and they release.

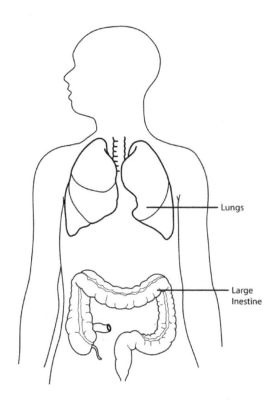

Lungs

Large Inestine

The Lungs receive chi from heaven and replenish us. The Lungs are the receivers of energy, taking it from the outside into ourselves. We receive on all levels, so we breathe emotionally and not just physically. In the Hindu tradition, the essence of breath is called prana which is of course analogous to the Chinese qi, and breath control is an important part of meditation techniques, where our breath is our connection to the universe. With each in-breath we take in energy from the universe, and with each out-breath we release toxic substances, creating space for new energy production.

If we follow thoughts of breathing a little further, we can imagine a couple of different sorts of people. In the first category are those who breathe in too much and breathe out too little. They strut around with inflated chests, they hold on tightly to what they have, and they cannot let go and relax. In the second category are those who breathe out more than they breathe in. Their chests are collapsed and they are continually lacking in energy. They constantly look needy.

The Large Intestine is rather like the dustbin man and its function is to store and dispose of waste. It can also be seen as the generator of evolution and change. If there is an imbalance in this organ then the rest of the system is put under strain, waste begins to accumulate and the other organs are put under more pressure. Symptoms such as feeling bloated, swelling, constipation, emotional 'stopping up', bad acne and boils, headache and stuffy nose, can all point to a Large Intestine imbalance. These descriptions are on a physical level, but the Large Intestine is seen as working on all levels of the body-mind-spirit. If a person is unable to let go then they will be constipated and stagnate on all levels, so the Large Intestine is just as important as the Lungs in terms of our 'connection to heaven' (heaven is a synonym for our mental and spiritual world). We can only grasp fresh ideas and think new thoughts if we can let go of mental waste and obsolete mind patterns. So on the mental level, the Large Intestine represents clarity of thought and the power of discernment, the striving for intellectual quality.

Since Metal represents our energetic connection with the universe, a Metal imbalance can show in a person as an inadequate bond to one's environment. Imagine a person who is lonely and withdrawn, who seems hard, cold and isolated from their surroundings. They show little feeling. These people have a Metal imbalance.

Sometimes the imbalance can show in people who have high ideals, striving for something that they can never achieve. Some may follow religion in a fixed and dogmatic way. They are intent on getting to heaven, know how to purify themselves, and want to convert others to their beliefs. However, and this is an important point, they are unable to let themselves go sufficiently to receive the spiritual quality of the essence of Metal. Too shallow breathing and too little excretion increase the desire for inner and outer purification, and we can think of cleanliness and hygiene fanatics, and highly dogmatic followers of a religion, as compensating for this Metal disturbance through their behaviour. Metal's striving for intellectual quality can turn into a rigid outlook, intolerant Puritanism, religious fanaticism, a type of spirituality that is lacking in enthusiasm or warmth, or spontaneity. These characteristics are typical of many religions, unfortunately.

The essence of Metal is not easy to deal with. Metal is concentration, letting go, grief, going within, leaving the world. At the same time Metal is our connection to the environment, to our vitality, to heaven. Often we need to go deeper within to perceive a deeper connection that is not visible in our daily lives. Only when we let go can a space be created in which the old can die and the new can be born, completing the circle. By letting go of our outer form our essence can be revealed.

Water: Vital Essence and Elimination

Water represents Winter: life has withdrawn into the ground, the power of life lies dormant in the seeds; we are in the period between death and rebirth. The characteristic of Water is sinking below, moving downwards, reaching the lowest level. Its energy is a vertical flow to the centre of the earth.

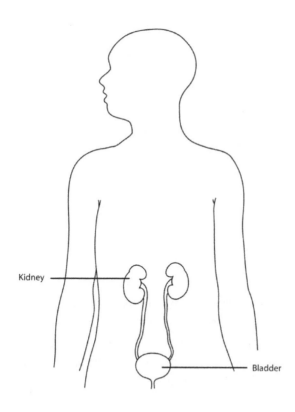

Fire draws up to the heavens and Water pulls us down to the depths, and on a spiritual level Water leads the soul and life back to its origins, to a deep consciousness, to the central core. "The river picks up the stream and leads it back to the sea".

In the body, Water manifests itself as the Kidneys and the Bladder, which - like all the 'organs' - are present at all levels of our body-mind-spirit.

The Kidneys are the storehouse of our vital essence, or basic constitution, something that we receive from our parents and our distant ancestors: our Ancestral Energy, an energetic 'genetic code' if you like.

Imagine the seed that represents the potential for development, compressed into a tiny space.

The Kidneys are the guardians of this essence. On a practical level, symptoms such as lethargy, a lack of acuity or perception, wishy-washy behaviour, and aching in the lower part of the abdomen, all point towards a lack of vital essence.

In Western medicine the Kidneys are responsible for dealing with water, which constitutes 65% of our body weight, and in Oriental medicine the Kidneys can be seen as the controller of the water supply in agricultural communities, a highly honoured position.

The Kidneys continually purify the organism through the filtration of water. They do not provide nourishment (Stomach and Pancreas), they do not supply us with life energy (Lungs), but there is no bodily function that cannot be carried out without water.

Water picks up waste products, prevents stagnation, it makes movement, freshness and the 'fluidity' of the body possible. The kidneys regulate the amount of water we have in our bodies and so a Kidney imbalance can show up in a variety of different ways, for example in swelling and bloating, difficulty in urinating, and inability to digest food.

Inner secretions require water, and digestion requires water when food is taken in and converted into a 'pulp' (this is where the phrase "Kidneys, Passage to the Stomach" comes from).

The Kidney is also referred to as the 'gateway to the stomach' because the vital essence is seen as contributing to the rotting and ripening function of the Stomach, the bringing to fruition and the assimilation. Thus the Kidneys support the stomach in its job.

Water moistens the body's orifices: the eyes, nose, mouth, ears, anus and sexual organs. It is necessary for temperature regulation - through perspiration - and for the maintenance of joint and muscle fluids.

The Kidneys are responsible for regulating the body's salts and minerals, and this hints at Water's connection with bones.

Our nervous system can only function properly when the body's fluids have the right composition of salts and minerals, and the proper functioning of our muscles depends on this too.

The brain and the spinal cord are in fact assigned to Water, and in ancient texts the brain is called the 'Sea of Marrow'. In Chinese medicine the Kidneys are considered as important as the Heart because they maintain the internal environment; the Kidneys are the basis of life.

TCM sees two distinct aspects of the Kidney: the yin-Kidney and the yang-Kidney, with the former corresponding the functions that we would be familiar with in Western medicine.

The yang-Kidney corresponds to the endocrine system: the adrenal glands, the sex glands, the islets of Langerhans in the Pancreas, the thyroid, the thymus and the pituitary.

Of the hormones produced by the adrenal glands, the androgens exert a direct effect on libido, and adrenaline, noradrenaline, cortisol and aldosterone regulate blood pressure and the balance of fluids in our body.

Interestingly, the adrenal glands produce hormones that mediate our fight-or-flight response: our biochemical response of fear, the emotion of Water.

The Bladder is not just seen as an organ of storage and elimination, but works with the Kidney in storing the vital essence. The Bladder is flexible and adaptable in its ability to store a little or a great amount without discomfort, and this flexibility and adaptability appears on all levels.

So someone who tends towards depression, or feels unable to cope with life situations, or someone who fears change, may have a Bladder imbalance.

Water holds the deepest secrets of life. When we accept the power of Water we become quiet inside and the surface of the lake becomes smooth. In this inner quiet, the world of dreams and the unconscious begins to open up.

Water is the element of the deepening of self and meditation. If one is at home in the depths then one can meet the storms on the surface calmly.

With Water - more than any other element - we come across that which has no name: the Tao.

Other Correspondences of the Elements

Each Element has associated with it a sense organ, a body part, an orifice, a physical manifestation, and a variety of other aspects, for example a colour, a taste, and a time of day.

An imbalance in an element can show itself as a characteristic symptom in one of these areas. In the following section I am just going to touch on a few of these.

Wood:

The Eyes are represented by Wood, so an eye problem could be associated with an imbalance in the Liver and Gall Bladder: blindness, short- or long-sightedness, astigmatism or any sort of distorted vision. These organs are associated with planning, judgement and decision-making, and you could say that it takes vision and sight to be able to make proper decisions.

Headaches at the crown, temples or behind the eyes are characteristic of Wood imbalance.

Since Wood governs cycles of growth, Wood imbalances can cause irregular or painful menstruation or premature birth, in growth disorders in childhood or puberty, and in cancer.

A healthy Wood element grows out in all directions, so imbalance may show itself in symptoms that only occur in one side of the body or in diseases where there is lack of co-ordination in the muscles, or glands or organs. Wood has an important role in co-ordinating the right and left hemispheres of the brain, and an imbalance can be expressed in psychiatric and neurological disorders, in Schizophrenia, and in some forms of epilepsy.

Finally, Wood is associated with the sound of Shouting, not surprising when you think of its connection with anger and aggression, so a person who always talks in a kind of shout, aggressive and forceful, is showing a Wood imbalance.

Fire:

The Ears are represented by Fire, and so the Heart, the Small Intestine, The Heart Protector and the Triple Heater are all involved in hearing. The Small Intestine would be involved in sorting sounds, and so ringing in the ears and deafness could be related to a Fire imbalance. These are more organic things, but a Fire imbalance could also be seen in someone who has difficulty in listening to others. Interestingly, the four Fire meridians are found near the ears.

The Tongue is the sense organ of Fire, so a speech impediment may be related to an imbalance in Fire, and this has already been discussed in more detail earlier. Fire also governs the maintenance and regulation of the entire circulatory system, so arteries and veins are the 'tissue' of Fire, and so are the Heart, Pericardium (the Western anatomical structure), the capillaries and all the hormones and regulatory mechanisms that are involved in the control of circulation. Thus an imbalance could be represented by hardening of the arteries, varicose veins, cold hands and thrombosis.

In ancient times the Pericardium was seen as an organ of Water, as a 'Yang-Kidney', and even now is seen as occupying a special central position between Kidney and Heart, between Water and Fire, between the upper and lower poles of a person. The significance of this is that in Chinese medicine it is seen as desirable to maintain a balance between left and right, above and below. In Western civilisation we have come to value the upper pole, to value Fires associations with love, speech and intellect. These are more treasured than the depths of Water, with its sexuality, meditation and sinking into the archaic levels of the soul. A balanced Pericardium forms a bridge between Water and Fire, allowing us to experience a fulfilled sexuality that brings forth joy and laughter. If the Pericardium is balanced, and chi can flow properly, then we feel a deep connection between sexual lust and love, and we are able to freely give and receive.

Though the Heart and Pericardium are both Yin organs, they are very different in their functions: the heart is responsible for inner matters like clarity of thought, speech, responsibility and motivation, whereas the Pericardium is responsible for blood circulation, heartbeat and heart rate on the physical level. Because of this, cold hands and feet are an indication of a lack of energy in the Pericardium, as is the person who has little warmth. Such people do not find much joy in sexuality, the stingy people who have a difficult time giving, people who need a long time to thaw, and closed people who do not laugh.

Earth:

Earth is represented by Flesh - the connective tissue and fat tissue - and a wasting disease may be due to an Earth imbalance. The state of the flesh reflects the Earth element. Earth also represents muscle. Since Earth is also related to the Mouth, many mouth diseases can be related to an Earth imbalance and practitioners of TCM can assess the condition of the Stomach and Spleen by looking at the lips.

Since Ideas and Opinions are associated with Earth, then someone who is displaying extreme dogmatism, or who is unable to create ideas or conclude thoughts, may have an Earth imbalance.

The colour yellow is associated with Earth, so if a person seems to have a subtle yellow hue coming from their face then this is indicative of an Earth imbalance. It is beyond the scope of this course to teach Oriental Visual Diagnosis, and it is unnecessary for our purposes.

Metal:

The Nose is associated with Metal, and so a limited or non-existent sense of smell can be associated with a Metal imbalance. The Chinese imagine an elemental spirit of Metal: an animal instinct that gives us the ability to 'smell' danger, to sense how other people are thinking and feeling about us, and to foresee future events. It is our sense of smell that allows us to differentiate between foods, people and surroundings that are good, or bad, for us. The connection with the Lungs is obvious and, interestingly, the Large Intestine Meridian is close to the nose.

A related correspondence is that of Mucus, and Metal governs the secretion of mucus by mucous membranes, and particularly in the breathing passages. So a dry throat, coughing etc. are associated with a Metal imbalance, as are a persistent nasal drip and blocked sinuses.

The themes of breathing, and the disposal of waste, are continued in Metal's association with the Skin. We are in contact with our environment through our skin, symbolic of the way that Metal connects us to the Universe. The skin is said to reflect the condition of the lungs, and it is not uncommon in Western medicine to see skin problems like eczema (skin problem) associated with asthma (lung problem). Psoriasis and rashes would be connected, as would acne, boils and pimples, which are all related to the accumulation of and getting rid of waste products through the skin. In a wider sense, we show our attitudes towards other people by allowing them to touch us, or by avoiding contact with them. We are 'in touch' with nature only as long as we enjoy the sensation of the wind, the coolness of water, the warmth of the sun and the feeling of the earth and plants.

The time of day for Metal is 0300 hrs - 0700 hrs. If we were to get up with the dawn, then this would be the time when we would start the day with some deep breaths, and defecation would take place quite naturally during these 'Metal' hours. Energy cultivation techniques like Tai Chi would be done in local parks when the sun is rising, in the fresh air.

Water:

The elemental spirit of Water is our will power, our will to survive, our sexual drive. It represents the vitality with which we master life. This spirit - called Zhen - can unfold when the organism is flowing freely, fresh and clean inside, and when the hormonal system is functioning effectively so the metabolism is finely tuned. In these circumstances power and vitality can develop. This power shows itself in supple body movements, flexible joints, sexual potency, strong bones and healthy teeth, a silky shine to the hair, good hearing, a tremendous urge for action and activity, and a healthy ability to adjust to the demands of circumstances.

Balance within Water depends on the relative strengths of the yin and yang Kidneys. When the yang energy is weak, or when the yin Kidney is relatively strong, then the will to live, vitality, and sexual drive decrease. The results may be a general weakness, impotence, frigidity and paralysing fear. When the yang Kidney is dominant then you may find a person who is constantly in a hurry, or a person who exhibits rigid behaviour and body movements. This rigidity shows itself mainly in the lower back, the sacro-iliac joints and the back of the legs (along the course of the Bladder meridian). Symptoms of this rigidity are such things as hollow back, disk problems in the lumbar area, sciatica, lumbago and bladder infections.

Other signs of a Water imbalance are kidney stones, kidney and urinary tract infections, bone diseases, loss of hair, some types of watery diarrhoea, menstrual disorders, insomnia, and constantly cold hands and feet.

In fact a lot of sexual functions depend on balance in Water: the health of reproduction and the workings of the testicles and ovaries for example.

The Ears are connected with Water, though we have already spoken about the effect of Fire, and the Small Intestine's sorting functions, on hearing. Water is more related to the sense organ itself and the semicircular canals. For this reason vertigo, lack of balance and dizziness can represent a Water imbalance, as well as middle ear infections.

The time of day for Water is 1500 hrs - 1900 hrs. A person with a Water imbalance might feel that this time of day is their best, when they feel more alive than usual, but more likely it might be the time of day when the person feels at their lowest ebb. There may also be an urgency to urinate during this period.

Five Element Theory: FAQ

How much theory do I need to be able to remember?

I want to say to you that the theory of the Five Elements is fascinating, but you can use this system effectively even if you know nothing at all about five element theory.

It is interesting to understand how a person's element imbalances are reflected in their mind/body/spirit, and it is satisfying to understand the changes that you see happening during a course of treatments, but that academic knowledge is not needed to use this system effectively... so don't get bogged down in the theory.

I am not an expert in Five Element theory, and you don't need to be either.

Experiencing the Five Energies

Five Element Symbols

I have channelled five symbols which represent energies that resonate at the characteristic frequencies of the five elements, and resonate strongly with the energies of each element's associated 'organs' and meridians.

The background to this is that I asked my spirit guide whether it would be possible to use symbols to represent the essence of the five elements and the response was positive. I asked if it would be possible for me to channel those symbols and the response was also positive.

I used 'automatic writing' and went through each element in turn, channelling each symbol a number of times to make sure that there was consistency in the way that it was being drawn out.

The symbols were consistent.

I then asked if using these symbols would produce greater treatment or healing benefits when compared with standard Reiki treatments. Obviously if the symbols produced no greater benefit than standard Reiki, there would be no point in continuing with them.

I received the message that these energies would indeed produce greater healing benefits than standard Reiki treatments. The reason for this is I believe that they focus the energy intensely on one particular aspect of a person - focusing on all the ramifications of an element, and because the focus is narrow, the effect is more intense.

You can see the same approach with the use of the standard Reiki symbols: as soon as you start using SHK for example, you are focusing intensely on mental/emotional balancing. Because you have narrowed the focus, you have intensified the healing effect.

Because the five element energies have so many ramifications, although the focus is narrow, the knock-on effects are many and varied, which is an interesting contradiction.

A Reiki Master and clairvoyant who had been helping me by giving me feedback about the symbols, energies and their effects had this to say after one of our 'experimentation' sessions:

"The energy I felt from the symbols made me very keen to continue learning more about them. It was so different from the traditional Reiki symbols and far more than I've felt from the other Seichim symbols I've been given (even though I've been 'attuned' to them)."
Chris Burns March 2001

The Fire Symbol

Start on the right and move to the left...

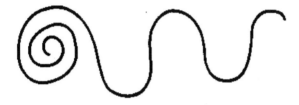

Colour: If you can see colours, you might imagine this symbol being drawn out in red.

The Earth Symbol

Draw a short line down, obliquely and to the left. Then make a sharp turn to the right and draw a line to the right, arcing anticlockwise in a full circle, then circling anticlockwise three times in a smaller circle that engulfs the original short oblique line.

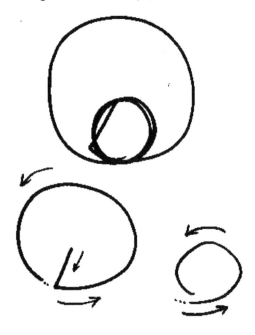

Colour: If you can see colours, you might imagine this symbol being drawn out in yellow.

The Metal Symbol

Start at the centre of the spiral, moving anticlockwise, spiralling outwards and plummeting to the ground. Then draw a straight line upwards obliquely to the right, level with the centre of the spiral.

Then draw a straight line upwards obliquely to the left. You are now at the top of the symbol. Follow this by tracing a triangle three times. The first stroke goes down and to the left, the second stroke goes horizontally to the right, and the third stroke goes vertically upwards. You finish at the pinnacle of the symbol.

Colour: If you can see colours, you might imagine this symbol being drawn out in white.

The Water Symbol

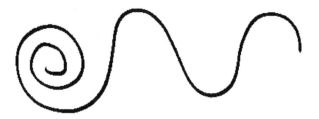

Start on the right and move towards the left.

The difference between the Fire symbol and the Water symbol as follows:

The Fire symbol is like a roller coaster. It falls down twice and then flies or leaps up into space, like flames licking at the sky.

The Water symbol falls down twice but then it stays down low, rolling out like a carpet or a wave, along the ground.

Colour: If you can see colours, you might imagine this symbol being drawn out in black.

The Wood Symbol

Draw a line vertically downwards. Then bounce up, over and to the left, curving round anticlockwise into the right-hand loop of what will be an 'infinity' symbol. Make the infinity symbol, left-right, left-right, left-right, so you have traced out three infinity symbols, finishing at the centre of infinity.

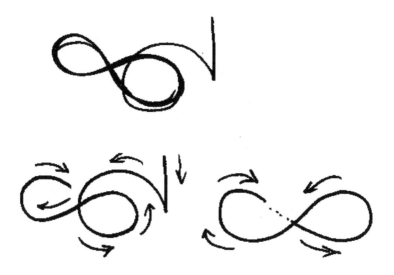

Colour: If you can see colours, you might imagine this symbol being drawn out in green.

93

Being attuned to these symbols

So long as you are already 'attuned' to Reiki, you can use these symbols and they will work for you.

You do not need to have been 'attuned' to these symbols for them to be effective. In fact, you do not need to be attuned to the Reiki symbols for them to work, either: so long as you are connected to Reiki – either through having received an attunement or an empowerment – then any symbol will focus the energy in a particular way without you having to go through a specific 'attunement' ritual.

The idea of attuning someone to a symbol before they can use it is a myth.

Five Element Energy Meditations

Introduction

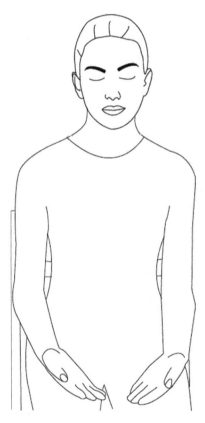

If you are going to be using the five elemental energies in practice – using them on yourself and using them on other people – then you should spend some time becoming thoroughly familiar with them.

Below you will see described some symbol meditations that you can use on a regular basis in order to 'become' or to 'assimilate' the five energies.

These are powerful meditations, and they have the potential to produce powerful effects within you. You can use the meditations in different ways:

You can if you like carry out a meditation for about 10 minutes daily, spending a couple of minutes experiencing each of the five energies, working in the order Wood Fire Earth Metal Water

Alternatively, you can if you like spend 5-10 minutes each day working with only one energy, for say 7-10 days. When you have completed 7-10 days of meditations using one energy, then spend a further 7-10 days using the next energy. Again follow the order Wood Fire Earth Metal Water

Technique

These meditations allow you to experience the distinctive qualities of each element. Try each approach and find out for yourself which variation feels more comfortable for you.

Meteditation #1

1. Sit with your eyes closed and your hands resting in your lap, palms uppermost.
2. Draw out the symbol in your mind's eye, up in the air above you.
3. Imagine cascades of energy flooding down onto you from the symbol.
4. Energy floods into your hands, into your head, into your torso.

Be aware of any sensations in your body, any impressions, any qualities you are experiencing. Where are the sensations located?

Be aware of your emotions, your thoughts, and your state of mind. Where is your attention directed?

Make notes afterwards on what you experienced.

Meditation #2

1. Sit with your eyes closed and your hands resting in your lap palms uppermost.
2. Draw out the symbol in your mind's eye, up in the air above you.
3. As you inhale, draw energy down from the symbol, into your crown.
4. Draw energy down the centre of your body to your Dantien *.
5. As you pause before exhaling, feel the energy get stronger in your Dantien.
6. As you breathe out, feel the energy spread through your body.

Be aware of any sensations in your body, any impressions, any qualities you are experiencing. Where are the sensations located? Be aware of your emotions, your thoughts, and your state of mind. Where is your attention directed? Make notes afterwards on what you experienced.

* The "Dantien" (Tanden in Japanese) is an energy centre that can be found two finger-breadths below your tummy button and 1/3rd of the way into your body. In Oriental thought it is seen as your personal energy reserve, the centre of your creativity and intuition, the seat of your soul. It is used extensively in energy cultivation techniques like Tai Chi and Chi Kung, in Martial arts, in creative pursuits and in the original form of Reiki!

Meditation #3

1. Sit with your eyes closed and your hands resting in your lap palms uppermost.
2. Draw out the symbol in your mind's eye, up in the air above you.
3. As you inhale, draw energy – AND THE SYMBOL - down into your crown.
4. Draw the energy – AND THE SYMBOL - down the centre of your body to your Dantien.
5. The symbol now resides in your Dantien
6. As you pause before exhaling, feel the energy get stronger in your Dantien.
7. As you breathe out, feel the energy spread through your body.
8. With the symbol remaining in your Dantien, repeatedly draw down and flood out energy in time with your breath

Be aware of any sensations in your body, any impressions, any qualities you are experiencing. Where are the sensations located?

Be aware of your emotions, your thoughts, and your state of mind. Where is your attention directed?

Make notes afterwards on what you experienced.

Feedback from 'Guinea Pigs'

What follows are some comments that were given to me by various people who I 'experimented' on. They drew the five energies into themselves, and gave me feedback on what they were feeling/experiencing.

Maybe some of their experiences tie in with what you have felt during your meditation on the energies. Try to give an explanation for their feelings based on your knowledge of the correspondences of the elements.

Meditating on Wood

Taggart
Contented happiness, balance, flexibility, 'inner smile', head wafting like a stem in a breeze randomly for a while until balance was achieved, toes and fingers tingling, heaviness or dull feeling in liver area.

Karen
Very relaxing, deeper breathing (not as deep as earth), softness, gentle warmth (not heat), pain in hairline, sensation in abdomen, soles of feet tingling, heel and foot more in contact with the ground.

Karen#2

Tingling from the knees to the feet. Downward movement from the knees to the feet. Pleasant. Drifting off. Took a long time before I felt anything.

Janet

Smooth, calm, feet fixed to the ground: rooted but not heavy... not pressure, top of body was more organic and flowing, calm breathing.

Christine

Beautiful. Feeling of physically swaying, blowing gently in the breeze. Gentle flowing resting at ears, breathing relaxed. Energy went to solar plexus and gently flowed. Circular movement in Dantien area. Very relaxing and gentle energy. Peace, calm, everything in the world is fine, is going to be fine, no fears, no anxieties. Being part of everything, grounded but in contact with the universe.

Hazel

Dependable. Soft. Safe. Drifting off to sleep. Soothing. Yellow/orange. Full of life, but not vibrant - a gentle, giving life. Not like earth though, not nurturing: contained life, capable of giving out. Inner strength.

Meditating on Fire

Taggart
Impassioned, extra positive outlook/feeling, arrogance, confidence, unsettled: wanting to get on and do things, many thoughts, progressive intense pressure in the heart area (not unpleasant) and tingling in abdomen, fast breaths, dry mouth, brightness, tingling ears, alertness, not sunk in chair as was the case with earth, full hands (not fizzing)

Karen
Bright orange colour, very swirly feeling, dry mouth, heaviness/pressure in heart, focused on the clock ticking like a heartbeat, faster shallower breathing and lots of breathing in, more aware of things outside - from my ears, not sunk into chair as was the case with earth.

Karen#2
Feeling down arms. Faster breathing. Alert. Poise. Lively feeling. Pressure by eyebrows (above, in the middle). Ready for action.

Janet
Heat in outer ear, sense of anger, energy movement in arms, not serene, shooting pressure across head.

Christine
Immediate warmth but a light feel, moving to the back/abdomen - a couple of inches above & below the

navel in the front and the back. A lot of expansion. Comforting yet invigorating within. Deep breathing. Felt good, open, aware, a loving energy.

Hazel
Prickly; jagged. Tingling in arms/shoulders. Almost vibratory, then feeling on cheekbones/tightening. Scalp tingling/standing on end. Intense. Back of skull sensation. No feeling of sinking down. Sitting up straight/upright. Very 'round the head'. Left with an 'alert' feeling. Didn't want to 'be one' with it. Feelings of positivity. Was 'in' the energy, but not part of it.

Meditating on Earth

Taggart
Deep muscular relaxation, dense heaviness, heavy limbs and body, connected-ness to the earth/roots/planet, thoughts of oneness, empty head, no thoughts, awareness of stomach (dull sensation) and spleen, slow deep breathing, fierce heat in hands

Karen
Green/brown colours, heat at back of neck and down back, blanket over shoulders and down the back, big releasing breaths, swirling/movement in head, empty head, slowed her down, deep breathing, wooziness.

Karen#2
Pleasantly tearful. Slowed breathing. Enveloped by cool green-ness. Still. Warm in stomach area. Shoulders going down. Sinking back into chair.

Janet
Heaviness in head, strong, thoughts of wholeness, feeling of lead, not uplifting but not oppressive.

Christine
Emerald green/yellow colour, energy in forehead base of skull. Travelled to upper chest and no further. Wobbly feeling; solid, tangible, heavy energy, moving with a 'ripple' effect. Calming and grounding.

Hazel
Shoulders relaxed. Energy washed down; leg dropped. Soft, gentle pressure, pushing me down. Warm & loving. Wonderful warm flow. Definitely a warm green colour. All encompassing. Stomach: everything settled (undulated, and then settled). Womb-like comforted feeling

Meditating on Metal

Taggart
Cool, reserved, analytical, detached, otherworldly, hardened attitudes, progressive heaviness in chest cavity and main part of abdomen, tingling in many areas of skin, tingling at sides of abdomen, fast shallow breath.

Karen
Cold nose, blue/white colour, shallow breathing, tingling/cold from the knees down, aware of nose/teeth/tongue, something totally alien, not organic, detachment, 'out of this galaxy' energy, not at all familiar, not welcoming, didn't embrace, just there - take it or leave it.

Karen#2
Cold. Tip of nose 'went'/pulsated. Hands cold. Sense of suspended time. Something close to face. Not pleasant: not unpleasant but not pleasant. Suspended: not thinking. Frozen. Came out of it easily. Absence of colour.

Janet
Rigid, immovable, heavy, sedated breathing because of great load on chest. Saw a symbol: vertical diamond with small square inside it, and four lines radiating off each side of the diamond.

Christine
Distinctive smell of metal filings, and a feeling of constriction in the chest, shallow breathing, suffocation. A very compressed energy. A straight rod going through spine, energy going out through the base of the spine. Feeling of wanting to take control, command, being overbearing, straight-laced. Hardened attitudes.

Hazel
Sharp, cutting, incisive. Very aware of a feeling in the crown (one of the points coming down). Symbol cut me down the middle, sharp, cold, incisive. Not threatened, but not comfortable either. Cutting to the essence, or the point of what is going on. Cuts through the crap. Feels 'sharper' afterwards. Odd.

Meditating on Water

Taggart
Heaviness in lower abdomen, or an awareness of that area, round to kidneys, contented shallow breathing, slow intermittent breaths, quiet serenity, tingling in inner ear, slow motion movements of the head for a while until it found a balanced position, balance, fluidity, cool gentle pulsing in hands

Karen
Something going on in the eyes (?bladder meridian), warming of the lower back, no colour, bladder awareness, movement down the legs, warm eyes, gentle, downwards sensations (not returning), not aware of breath, feeling between the shoulder blades, creeping awareness of lower abdomen, heaviness.

Karen#2
Sleepy. Aware of nose/tip. Didn't want to open eyes. Slow, woozy (not unpleasant). Befuddled. Intense urge to drink water. Difficult to find words. No particular colour: pale. Need to go to the loo.

Janet
Pressure inside ears, calm, soft balls of energy in hands, tingling in back of head, calm unforced breathing.

Christine

Energy passed to third eye and throat and became ice cold, moving down arms, flowing down back and out through feet. Feeling quite emotional.

Hazel
Need to go to the loo. Woozy. Slowly a feeling starting at the lower back and then movement, smooth, going down the legs and out, one leg (L) more than the other. Cold legs/feet. A 'clearance': feeling soft, swirly. Heat in a wonky knee. Intense thirst.

"I started with wood, I could see young trees with my inner eyes. Then I switched to fire, and wow! I felt like I was surrounded by huge flames, warming me very quickly and completely. I felt a slight pressure on my heart, and my heartbeat increased. After that, I changed to Earth, it was a very comfortable, nurturing feeling, the energy went into my stomach and was very calming there (I am having a lot of digestion problems at the moment, due to a change of my diet). I then channelled Metal, which felt kind of cold, strange, light, it started activating my kidneys. This activation became very strong when I finally channelled Water, it felt like a hot water bottle on my lower back, very nice and warm, activating and energising my kidneys"
Stefanie, Germany

Working on
Your Self

Monitoring the State of Your Elements

So, you know about the Five Elements and how they relate to your physical, mental and emotional states, you have looked at and explored five symbols that you can use to experience the five different energies and you have started to experience the five energies through meditation.

Now we are going to move on to something that I find exciting: being able to intuit the state of your elements: to discover which hold too much chi, which hold too little, and which seem just fine.

You may not realise it just yet, but you already know the state of your elements.

All the information and insights that you need are already there, within you.

You may be able to access these insights easily and effortlessly or you may need to practise before you feel comfortable with trusting what is coming to you.

Intuitive knowledge can come to people in a whole range of different ways. For some, they just 'know' what their elements are doing.

For others, the information pops up in one of many different forms: a word, a sound, a feeling or an image.

Some people need a bit more 'structure' in order to access what is already within them, and they can use different 'props'.

A prop might be a weight dangling on a string – a pendulum - or some other 'already set up beforehand' physical movement.

A prop can also involve using a visual image in your mind's eye, where they way that the image changes or moves or presents itself provides you with the information that you need.

'In your head' ways of accessing intuitive knowledge are usually more speedy and versatile than physical-based methods.

For example, if you're using a pendulum you have to keep on opening your eyes, picking it up and putting it down, whereas if you're doing it all 'in your head' then you can perceive the state of your elements in real time, instantly, 'on the fly'.

Your Goal

Your goal should be to end up able to sense the state of your elements without having to resort to a physical prop, though they can be useful to begin with to help build your confidence and to give you an opportunity to practise being in an 'accessing intuition' state of mind.

You will find lots of different options and variations described below.

Try them out and see what works best for you. Every time you try one you are practising getting your head into the right sort of state to access what you already know on some level.

General impressions: an "inner knowing"

Let's start with a simple opening-to-intuition meditation and we can find out what your subconscious is going to provide you with. This is what you can do:

Sit quietly with your eyes closed and take a long, deep breath. Imagine any stress or tension just drifting out of you as you exhale.

Be still.

Now focus your attention on your Liver and Gall Bladder; you know where they are in your body. You are noticing the state of the Wood element in you.

Maybe remember how the Wood energy feels, or bring to mind the Wood symbol, to focus your attention on that energy. Just become that energy for a time.

Be still with these organs and this element and be aware of any impressions that you might have.

Maybe you might have a word come to mind, or a feeling, an image of some word or an "inner knowing" about the state of this element.

Does it hold too much chi at the moment?

Is its energy depleted in some way?

Or does it seem fine, balanced, perfectly appropriate for you?

Take your time.

Make a note of what impression you have: too much, too little, or just fine.

Then move on to the element of Fire, focusing your attention on your Heart and Small Intestine. Maybe remember how the Fire energy feels, or bring to mind the Fire symbol, to focus your attention on that energy.

Move through the other elements - Earth, Metal and Water - making notes on your impressions each time.

You may find that the state of these elements is quite clear to you straight away; if so, congratulations!

It can be surprising sometimes how quick, how immediate the response can be: as soon as you ask the question, the answer is there!

It doesn't have to be difficult.

Or you might find that this takes a bit of practice, and what you are practising is tuning into yourself, noticing your energies, how they feel, their strength or weakness or 'just-fine'-ness.

What happened during these exercises?

Were your impressions coming through to you in a fairly standard way, with a particular word or image or sensation or feeling each time, or did it seem quite random?

You might find that your subconscious mind has showed you, through this exercise, its 'default' way of displaying or providing the information to you.

Or maybe you might find that you have an image of each element which alters in some way, depending on what sort of state it is in.

You shouldn't put up any barriers or expect your intuition to come to you in any particular way.

Try this exercise later on, and on a different day, and see what happens.

Dowsing - General

If you are going to treat yourself, it will be useful if you can see the effect of the self-treatments on your elemental imbalances from day to day. A simple and effective way of doing this is by dowsing: using a pendulum.

Not everyone gets on well with a pendulum, but it's a useful skill to have if it 'clicks' with you, and you can use it as a stepping-off point, to build your confidence in your intuitive ability and to get you use to 'tuning in' to your intuition, before going freestyle and intuiting purely in your head.

In this section I'm going to talk about using a pendulum in general – the basic principles – and then I move on to show you how to use a pendulum to look at the state of your elements in quite a precise way.

Introduction

You can use anything that dangles as a pendulum, whether it be a crystal, a ring or a piece of plastic, but pendulums are not expensive and the easiest to use would be lightweight metal pendulums: I have a nice brass pendulum on a chain. Some use crystals suspended by a thread but they are not so robust.

'Yes' and 'No' Answers

The first thing to do is to find out how your pendulum is going to interact with you: what movements it is going to make for different responses.

You need to know what it is going to do to show you a 'yes' or 'no' answer. Try asking 'am I a man?' or 'am I a woman?'

Blank your mind for a few moments, hold the pendulum away from your body, suspending it between your thumb tip and index fingertip, relax, and see what it does.

Don't rest your elbow on your leg or the arm of a chair because the pendulum won't give you a strong response: your muscles need room to move it!

For me, 'yes' is a clockwise movement and 'no' is side-to-side, but it seems to vary from one person to another. You could try saying 'show me your yes response' and 'show me your no response' and see what happens.

If you try asking 'what should I do now' then you may elicit a response that means ' I can't answer that question with a yes/no', or 'that is a stupid question'.

This is a useful response to have, actually, since otherwise you are limiting the pendulum to a 'yes' or 'no' response, neither of which may always be the appropriate answer!

You can interpret the 'stupid question' response as meaning 'you need to re-phrase your question before I can answer it properly'.

The 'Neutral' position

I have found that it is easier for the pendulum to give you answers quickly if it is already moving, rather than holding it still every time, whereupon it has overcome inertia every time it answers you.

In my case, I continually swing the pendulum forwards-and-backwards as a 'neutral' position before asking the questions, because that motion is different from my 'yes', 'no' and 'stupid question' responses.

Obtaining 'Permission'

Various books recommend that you ask a few questions before entering upon a new endeavour, as follows:

1. Can I do this? (Am I able to do this?)
2. Should I do this? (Is it right or appropriate for me to do this?)

3. May I do this? (simply politeness really)

If you get 'yes' responses to all the questions then you can go ahead.

Another approach could be to ask (thanks to Tina Shaw):

1. Can I? (Do I have the skill?)
2. May I? (Do I have permission, or is it appropriate?)
3. Am I ready? (Am I appropriately prepared for this, have I considered all I need to consider?)

If any of the answers are 'no' then do not try any more at that time. You do not have to go through this procedure every time you use a pendulum, only when you are intending to use a pendulum in a different way, or for a different purpose, than you have before.

Dowsing Chakras

Dowsing the state of someone's chakras is not something that you do when carrying out Five Element Reiki, and not something that you need to do when practising standard Reiki, but it is a useful exercise to carry out in order develop your skills with the pendulum.

Ask 'am I able to use this pendulum to dowse the state of a person's chakras?' If you get a 'yes' response then you can ask these questions:

- What will you show me if the chakra is open?
- What will you show me if the chakra is closed or spinning sluggishly?
- What will you show me if the chakra is spinning too fast?

For me, the responses are my 'yes', 'no' and 'stupid question' responses.

If you were going to experiment on yourself, just sit quietly and focus your attention on your crown chakra. Get your pendulum moving (if you have a convenient 'neutral' movement) and say to yourself 'show me the state of my crown chakra'; see what the pendulum does.

Then move on to the third eye, throat etc. all the way to the root chakra.

Do this on different days and notice if there are any changes. You are just flexing your intuitive 'muscles', getting used to clicking into a receptive state of mind.

If you are experimenting on someone that you are going to be treating, and they are lying on a treatment table, do this: before you start the treatment, hold the pendulum so that it dangles over the crown chakra, say to yourself 'show me the state of the crown chakra', and see what the pendulum does.

Then move on to the third eye, throat etc. all the way to the root chakra.

Make a note and then repeat the process at the end of the treatment to see what difference there is.

In fact you do not have to dangle the pendulum over each chakra; you can happily dowse the chakras standing by the person's side.

You do not have to have the subject in the same room as you, either, so you can dowse the state of their chakras before they arrive for the appointment!

Within the world of dowsing, it is common for the dowser to have some sort of 'witness' - for example a lock of the person's hair, by way of making a definite connection with the person about whom they are seeking information.

I have not felt the need to do this with Reiki clients, so I believe that Reiki and intent is connection enough.

Common Chakra 'presentations'

I have found that it is quite common for the throat, heart and solar plexus chakras to be closed, which ties in with inability to express oneself and current/long term emotional issues respectively.

I found a closed root chakra in a girl with anorexia and a woman with multiple addictions.

I found fast-spinning third eye chakras in a counsellor, research chemist, a molecular geneticist and web consultant.

This book isn't about Chakras, though, so if you are interested and want to learn more, there are many books on the subject.

Practice

Practise using a pendulum in this way until you feel comfortable with it, and then you can move on to the next section, where you will find out how to dowse the state of your elements with a great deal of precision.

The 'coin toss challenge'

From Tina Shaw:

"This is scary because you can fail but there is no such thing as failure - only feedback - and this is particularly true of learning to work intuitively.

Have a partner toss a coin 10 times and each time they look at the result and write it down.

You on each occasion use your pendulum to identify whether it's heads or tails.

If you have scored 7 out 10 correct then you've got some pretty good dowsing skills and what a confidence boost!

There is no way to positively prove your results when doing energy work and the good thing is that you know the energy will work for the highest good of the person regardless, but building confidence in your ability to dowse or intuit does empower your work greatly.

The learning that you can obtain from this exercise is when you've got it wrong: what did you notice within yourself - did your inner voice or vision tell you the correct result and the pendulum didn't, was your question or intention a little off or was your mind over thinking?

Dowsing is a great teacher of mindfulness because we can get in the way of the results if we are not mindful."

How to Dowse your Elements

Dowsing someone's Elements: basic method

To start dowsing the elements, you could ask these simple questions. Starting with Wood:

Is my Wood in balance?
If YES, then you can move on to the next element

In NO, Wood is not in balance, you need to ask a further question...

Is there too much chi in my Wood?
If YES, ask a supplementary question:
Does Wood hold the greatest excess of chi of all the elements for me? If YES, keep a note of that.

If NO, there is not too much chi in Wood, then Wood must be deficient in chi. Ask a supplementary question: does Wood hold the greatest deficiency of chi of all the elements for me? If YES, keep a note of that.

Now you can move on to the next element. Use whatever order you like, but going from Wood - Fire - Earth - Metal - Water will help to reinforce the nourishment cycle in your mind!

Using this sequence you can find out which elements - if any - are already in balance, which elements hold an excess or deficiency of chi, and which two elements hold the greatest excess and the greatest deficiency in chi.

Dowsing someone's Elements: precise method

There is a way of being more precise than this, though. Using a pendulum, it is possible to find out in detail about the degree of imbalance of all your elements.

You can find out which elements are balanced, which elements hold too much chi, which elements are deficient, and the degree to which they are deficient or in excess.

By using a semicircular 'scale' – a bit like a protractor - with arbitrary percentages from 0% - 100%, it is possible to find out, say, that Wood has a 20% excess of chi while Fire has a 60% deficiency etc.

This is useful information because:

1. You can compare the relative imbalances of all the elements.
2. You can see how an imbalance in one element is reflected in imbalances in the supporting or controlling elements.

3. You can monitor your own progress more accurately, and see how the elements change in relation to each other from one self-treatment to another.

Technique

Look at the 'Dowsing Grid', which you will find below and in the Appendix. Zero is represented by a vertical line running up the page. To the right you can see a scale running as far as +100, in increments of 20 points, which represents elements that are holding too much chi. To the left you can see a scale running as far as -100, in increments of 20 points, which represents elements that are deficient in chi.

You can use this grid to simply and quickly find out about the state of each element: whether it is in balance, and if it is out of balance, whether it contains too much or too little chi, and to what degree.

This is what you do:

1. Hold the pendulum with its point hovering over the midpoint of the baseline, the point from which the 'spokes' radiate, or set it moving along the 'zero' line, in 'neutral'.

2. Say "Show me the state of my Wood element". Maybe remember the Wood energy that you

have experienced before, or bring to mind its
symbol.

3. See in what direction the pendulum swings.

If the pendulum swings vertically up & down the page,
forwards and backwards, then the element is in balance.

If the pendulum swings to the right then the element
contains too much chi; record the degree of excess to
the nearest 10 points. If the pendulum swings to the left
then the element contains too little chi.

Record the degree of deficiency to the nearest 10
points. You do not need absolute precision and the
numbers are not empirical anyway. They are just a
guide.

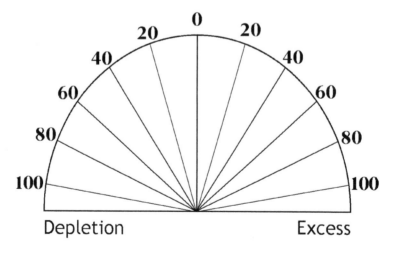

Students talk about balance and imbalance

"After doing Hsin Tao, the self-healing technique used by Shaolin monks, a couple of weeks ago I had a massive clearing - the worst migraine I have ever experienced. It concerned me so much that I knew finally had to get to the bottom of the cause of my migraines/headaches. So I sought the help of an acupuncturist. It is fascinating to watch her work and talk to her about the Five Elements. Using your methods I had already detected major imbalances in my Wood, Earth & Fire which she confirmed."
Jeannie, England

"A strange thing. I worked really hard on myself last evening and I touched zero i.e. balanced chi, on 2 of the elements. I was stunned, and yet wasn't surprised. Strange. I felt very neutral in many ways and getting near neutrality allowed so much clarity."
Ipsita, England

"I am in balance! Feels great too."
Ellen, England

"Couldn't believe it today when I started to detect my energy imbalances I found they were all in balance. Such a joy because I have been working so hard towards achieving this. Even if I find tomorrow there is a

slight imbalance at least I know it is possible! Needless to say I feel wonderful...."
Jeannie, England

"The day before yesterday, my 10th day of self-treatment, I touched zero on all 5 elements. I stared and stared, not unbelieving, but just.....stared."
Ipsita, England

Using Visualisation to Intuit your Elements

Using a pendulum, using muscle movements, isn't the only way of accessing intuitive knowledge. We can use creative visualisation to access our intuition, and this can be quicker than using a 'prop' and waiting for muscle movements to jiggle a crystal on a string.

I am going to run through some variations in this section.

Using an imaginary pendulum

We have just been talking about using a pendulum, so let's try using an imaginary one!

You might be surprised how straightforward it is for you to move from a real pendulum to an imagined one because the intuitive information that you are accessing is just the same; you are just altering a little bit the method that your subconscious is using to present it to you.

So, bring out your imaginary pendulum in your mind's eye and notice how it appears to you, its size and shape, length and weight, its density or physical 'presence'.

Practise moving it in different ways: front and back, side to side, clockwise, anti-clockwise. Feel its 'density'. You need to start by obtaining 'permission' to use the pendulum (see "Dowsing – general" above) and ask questions to establish what its 'yes', 'no' and 'stupid question' responses will be.

Don't assume that your imaginary pendulum is going to move in the same way as the physical one you have been using. This is a new pendulum!

Play around with this and see what's possible for you.

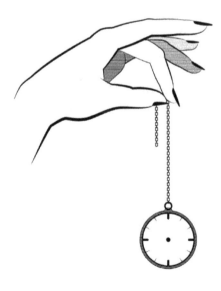

Using imagined text

OK, let's move away from things that are swinging, whether for real or in our imaginations, and let's take a look at things that might just pop up in your mind's eye. An intuitive method that works well for some people is to use words, written out in one's mind's eye, and notice what happens to those words and what meaning that might convey to us.

Try looking at the words for Wood, Fire, Earth, Metal and Water in turn, in your mind's eye. Like this:

Wood   Fire   Earth   Metal   Water

Intend that these words represent the state of your elements.

Look at each word in turn, or you might notice one or two that just jump out at you straight away.

You might notice that one word stands out as larger, or in **bold type**, or in a *different font* or in a **different colour**.

One word might be smaller than the rest.

The element or elements that stand out like this are the ones that need your attention.

Maybe you can't see a different font or size, or boldness... but maybe one of the words is buzzing or jumping up and down or is in a different colour, maybe a word is flashing on and off or seems so much heavier than the others, while another word wants to sail off like a helium balloon.

I do not know what your word images will do to indicate the state of an element, so you will need to experiment and discover for yourself what your personal 'code' is.

Can you tell whether an element has too much chi or too little chi by the way its word appears to you?

Compare the results of this way of intuiting with the results that you get from using a real or imagined pendulum. How do they compare?

Using an imaginary 'slider'

You can obtain the same answers that a pendulum might give you by using a constructed visual image, something that you bring to existence in your mind's eye.

What I like to use is an imaginary 'slider'. You have probably seen sliders in photos of recording studios, where they have banks of dozens of them on mixing desks, controlling volume and other effects

You can bring into your mind's eye a single sliding scale, either running horizontally or vertically. I use them vertically because that's how they look in real life. I find sliders to be really versatile. You may find that too, or you may not like them.

So, here you can see a vertical scale. Imagine that at the top of the scale lies the answer 'yes' and at the bottom lies the answer 'no'.

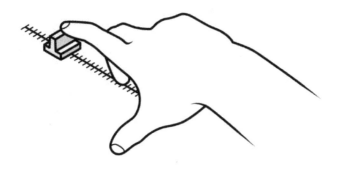

Imagine that the slider is at the very middle point of the scale to begin with.

Ask a question and see where the slider goes: to the top or the bottom. If the slider stays in the middle, maybe vibrating or jiggling in an uncertain fashion, that means that it is unable to answer the question, or you need to rephrase the question somewhat.

You can use this slider in exactly the same way that you can use a real or imagined pendulum.

But we can also use this sort of visualisation to be very precise about intuiting the state of our elements, by using an imaginary 'mixing desk'. Here's how…

The imaginary 'Mixing Desk'

A method that I use to look at the state of the elements is to visualise a 'mixing desk' like they have in a recording studio, with five different sliders, and you can see a cartoon of one of those below:

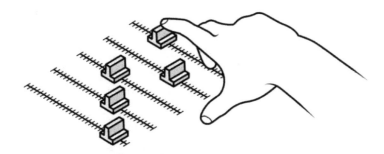

Each slider has a little knob that slides up and down the vertical track. One slider is for each element, arranged from left to right in this order: Wood, Fire, Earth, Metal, Water.

If the slider is at the very top of its track then it represents a 100% excess of chi. If the slider is at the very bottom of its track then this represents a 100% deficiency of chi.

If the slider is smack bang in the middle of its track, and you could imagine a little 'click' sound as it rests there, then the excess or deficiency is 0%: the element is in balance.

Now, if the slider is ¼ of the way between 0 and +100% then there is 25% excess, if it is half way between 0 and −100% then there is 50% deficiency.

This is what you can do:

Using five sliders next door to each other

1. Bring into your mind's eye an image of the 'mixing desk' with its five sliders, going from left to right displaying Wood, Fire, Earth, Metal and Water, one slider for each element.

2. Say "Show me the state of my Wood element". Maybe remember how the Wood energy feels, or bring to mind the Wood symbol, to focus your attention on that energy. Just become that energy for a moment.

3. See what happens to the first slider, on the far left.

4. If it stays where it is and does not move, maybe making a little clicking sound, then that element is in balance. If it slides up then there is an excess of chi in that element. If it slides down there is a deficiency of chi in that element. The distance it travels shows you the amount of the excess or deficiency. You could even 'zoom in' in your mind's eye and imagine 10% increments,

like a thermometer scale. Where does the slider stop? What is the percentage?

5. Write it down.

6. Now move on to the next slider, the one for Fire. Maybe remember how the Fire energy feels, or bring to mind the Fire symbol, to focus your attention on that energy. The slider starts on the 'balance' point, half way up. See where it slides; see where it stops. What is the percentage?

7. Now follow this procedure for the other three elements: Earth, Metal and Water.

Using only one slider to find the answers

Having five sliders might be a bit challenging or confusing. If that is the case, just use a single slider, which you re-use!

1. Bring into your mind's eye an image of the 'mixing desk' with its SINGLE slider. You are going to start by looking at your Wood element.

2. Say "Show me the state of my Wood element". Maybe remember how the Wood energy feels, or bring to mind the Wood symbol, to focus your attention on that energy. Just become that energy for a moment.

3. See what happens to your slider and write down the result.

4. Now use your slider to look at the state of Fire. The slider starts on the 'balance' point, half way up. Say "Show me the state of my Fire element". See where it slides; see where it stops. What is the percentage? Write it down.

5. Now follow this procedure for the other elements.

Using Physical Movements to Intuit your Elements

Not everyone gets on well with visualising things, though it has to be said that you don't need to be able to visualize things very well: even a fuzzy, dim image works perfectly well; images don't have to be in perfect focus or in Technicolor!

In fact, a lot of people who think that they 'don't visualise very well' don't realise how badly everyone can visualise things! Visual memory and visual images are a bit like the images that cameras on the first mobile 'phones produced: grainy and a bit rubbish!

In any case, not being able to visualise, or worrying about whether you can visualise well enough, won't hold you back in terms of intuition because you can use physical versions of the visual images if you like. I shall explain.

If you have trained with Reiki Evolution at Second Degree, you will be familiar with 'Reiji ho', the intuitive method where you allow the energy to move your hands, which drift with the energy to the right place to treat. Sometimes people find that the energy causes their hands to drift away from the body, sometimes quite a distance, to say 1-2 feet away.

So you know that the energy, or your intuition or your subconscious mind, is able to control muscles and direct movements of your hands and arms if you allow it to.

Your physical slider

Imagine that you are holding a credit card between your thumb and bent index finger – the card is horizontal – rather like you were just about to slide the card into the slot in a cash machine.

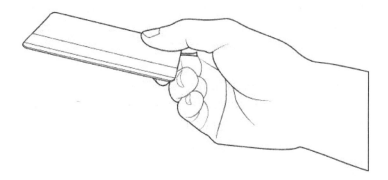

Alternatively, you can imagine that you are holding a pen or conductor's baton between your thumb and index finger:.

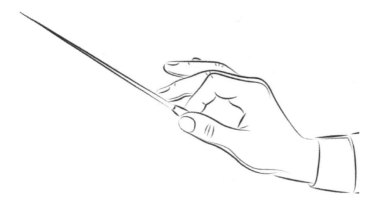

Either of these is your physical 'slider'.

You are going to imagine that there is a vertical scale that your hand/slider can move up and down. You start with your hand in what seems like is the middle of the scale: a comfortable position to hold.

Say to the slider "please slide to the top of the scale"; your hand should move upwards and then stop (mine moves up by about 9 inches).

Then return the slider to its centre 'stop' and ask the slider to slide down to the bottom of the scale; your hand should move downwards and then stop.

If the slider moves ridiculously far up and down, just tell it that it is too long and show it, by moving your hand, where the top and bottom points should be.

Now you have your physical slider which you can use instead of imagining a visual image.

You can also use your slider in two ways:

As a 'yes/no' scale

This is rather like dowsing with a pendulum. "YES" is at the top of the scale, "NO" is at the bottom, and if the slider hovers in the middle then it can't answer your question in a YES/NO fashion.

As a graduated scale

Here you can have +100% at the top, -100% at the bottom and 0% at the centre point of the scale.

Start with the slider at that centre point, half way along the scale.

A question like, "show me the state of my Earth element" will cause the slider to move up or down the scale to the relevant percentage, to show an excess or deficiency of chi.

Five Element Self-Treatments

The five element energies, and knowledge of their corresponding 'organs', can be used for self-development and balancing.

When you learn standard Reiki healing, often you are just given one self-treatment method: these are the hand positions; this is what you do.

On Reiki Evolution First Degree courses we try to be more flexible than that by providing students with a range of self-treatment methods: some entirely meditative, some involving 'hands-on' and some intuitive.

We do this so students can experiment and explore different methods to find what approaches work best for them.

So In this section I'm going to show you a whole load of Five Element self-treatment variations, starting with some gentle self-treatment methods, and then moving on to more potent or focused variations.

You should experiment to see what suits you best, or use different approaches on different occasions, as feels appropriate.

The 'bare bones' of self-treatments

In all of these variations, you are going to be either

1. Visualising something
2. Using "hands-on"

And you can self-treat very gently, or you can make things more intense by using symbols and your intuition.

The simplest Five Element self-treatment...ever!

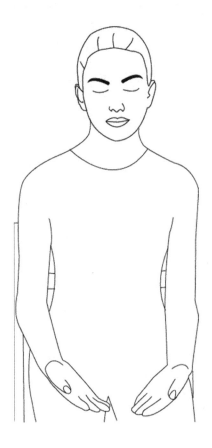

I thought we could begin with what is probably the simplest way possible of carrying out a Five Element self-treatment. You don't visualise anything, you don't use your hands for anything, and you don't use a symbol or imagine anything happening. You just sit and allow Reiki to balance your elements.

Basically, all you do is set your intent, sit, and let it happen!

Here's what to do…

Begin by sitting comfortably in a chair with your eyes closed and your hands resting in your lap, palms uppermost.

Close your eyes and take a couple of long deep breaths to settle yourself. Say to yourself "I am now going to bring my elements into balance".

Focus your attention on your Tanden, that energy centre just below your navel and 1/3rd of the way into your body. It's always a good idea to centre and ground yourself by focusing for a moment on this, the centre of your personal universe.

Your intention here is to receive sufficient energy to produce balance in your elements, by the energies boosting any elements that are depleted.

Your intention is also that if there is too much Chi in an element, the energy will put your body in a space where it can dissipate the energy, and will not exacerbate the imbalance.

Your intention is that the energies will bring into balance all the various correspondences of each element, not just the physical organs, which are just a small part of what each element represents.

So three intentions here: (1) boost depleted elements, (2) allow 'excess' elements to dissipate their excess, and (3) balance physical, mental, emotional and spiritual aspects of each element.

Just sit quietly and allow the energy to do what it needs to do to bring your elements into balance, and when you feel that the session is over for today, just take a long, deep breath, bring yourself back and open your eyes.

This meditation is a variation on my "simplest self-treatment method ever", which I describe in my book, "Liberate Your Reiki!" and can also be found on the Reiki Evolution web site, as a blog post.

Self-treatment through breathing light

You know that each element has an associated colour, and what we are going to do with this meditation is to flood that associated colour through the 'organs' that relate to each element.

The elements come in pairs, as you know, with one solid organ and one hollow organ. We will flood the solid organ with colour first, and then flood that colour into the related hollow organ.

When we do this, we will imagine a bright, intense and powerful light, one that cleans and clears and cleanses.

We will time this flooding of colour with our in-breath and our out-breath, breathing the intense, bright colour into the organ on the in-breath and then on the out-breath we will flood the light out of our bodies to the universe.

So you can see this meditation as a variation on 'Joshin Kokkyu ho' (soul cleansing breathing method) where you breathe energy into a part of your body and then breathe the energy out to the universe.

And of course, because you are attuned to Reiki, the energy will 'click in' and follow the passage of light that you are imagining, framing itself in such a way that it represents the quality of light you are working with, resonating at the frequency of the corresponding element, 'organs' and meridians.

As the light flows out of us, by the way, we will notice that the light has become stale, cloudy or dull, as it removes any 'impurities', and in particular as it takes away any negativity from the emotion that is associated with that element.

And in fact you could, if you liked, use your perception of the dullness or dirtiness of the expelled light as a guide to how long to work on that element, so that you carry on with the breathing cycle for that element until you perceive the light as becoming clean and clear.

In many relaxation-style meditations, it is not uncommon for people to progressively relax their bodies starting with the upper part of the body, moving along the torso to the legs, and in this meditation we will echo that by starting to work on the most highly-placed 'organ' in our bodies (the Lungs), then moving down through the Heart, Spleen, Liver and Kidneys.

Take a look at this list, which reminds you of the elements, organs and related colour:

Element	Solid Organ	Hollow Organ	Emotion	Colour
Metal	Lung	Large Intestine	Grief	White
Fire	Heart	Small Intestine	Joy	Red
Earth	Spleen	Stomach	Pensiveness	Yellow
Wood	Liver	Gall Bladder	Anger	Green
Water	Kidneys	Bladder	Fear	Deep Blue

What to do

Begin by sitting comfortably in a chair with your eyes closed and your hands resting in your lap, palms uppermost.

Close your eyes and take a couple of long deep breaths to settle yourself. Say to yourself "I am now going to clear and cleanse my elements, and release any negativity from my emotions".

As in the previous meditation, focus your attention on your Tanden, that energy centre just below your navel and 1/3rd of the way into your body. It's always a good idea to centre and ground yourself by focusing for a moment on this, the centre of your personal universe.

Imagine the source of Reiki above you, the source of a brilliant white light which is flooding down to you.

1. As you breathe in, the bright white light floods into and fills your lungs. The light is strong, intense, powerful and clears and cleanses the whole of your lungs.

2. As you pause before exhaling, the bright light floods into your large intestine, clearing and cleansing that organ too.

3. As you breathe out, the white light floods out of you to the universe, taking with it any impurities and releasing any negativity from the emotion of Metal.

4. Repeat this cycle of in-breath and out-breath until you feel that enough has been achieved for this session, or until the light you are expelling has become clean and clear.

Now move on to repeat the process for Fire, breathing into and out of the Heart and Small Intestine.

Continue to follow the same process for Earth, Wood and Water.

Remember that you are not hyperventilating here; that is not the purpose of the exercise. You are moving light – moving energy – in time with your gentle, normal breath.

If you wish to work further with the emotions of anxiety and anger (two emotions that feature strongly in the Reiki precepts!) I have created something called "The Releasing Exercise" for you, which I describe in my book, "Liberate Your Reiki!" and which can also be found on the Reiki Evolution web site, as a blog post.

"Gentle" self-treatments

I see these gentle Five Element self-treatments as a way of nudging the elements into balance, and then going on to send the energy deeper and deeper into each element and its correspondences, bringing each element into balance on all levels: in terms of the physical body, in terms of mental states and emotions and in terms of spiritual aspects.

In our self-treatments, we will be going through each element in turn, drawing its energy into the element's organs. We will follow this order:

Wood, Fire, Earth, Metal, Water

This sequence follows the flow of the seasons through the year, starting with the expansion and new growth of spring and moving on to the intensity of summer. Summer leads on to the 'pause' of Indian Summer, which the leads to the contraction of autumn and the still waiting period of winter.

We will follow that sequence through our bodies by using the five element energies in that same order.

Intuiting the state of your elements

This way of self-treating does not require you to intuit the state of your elements, by the way, though it would be really interesting to keep an eye on what's happening with them; that would also be good practice for you in flexing your intuitive muscles.

Which intuitive approach should you use? Whichever one feels most comfortable for you.

Use one of these self-treatment methods each day for a couple of weeks and keep notes on the changes in your elements each day.

How long to spend on each element?

I suggest below that you spend a few minutes on each element. If you were to spend 3 minutes on each one, you would have carried out a self-treatment lasting for 15 minutes, which is a good amount of time for a self-treatment session, I think.

But if you know the state of your elements, and one or two are particularly out of balance, it makes sense to spend a bit longer treating those elements, and a bit less time working on the others. You should treat the elements that are in balance too, a little bit. Be guided by the state of your elements.

Gentle 'Hands On' Self-Treatment method

For this gentle hands-on self-treatment method, you can either sit on a chair or lie down on a treatment table. Close your eyes and take a couple of long deep breaths to settle yourself.

Say to yourself "I am now going to bring my elements into balance". Your intention here is to receive sufficient energy to produce balance in your elements, by the energies boosting any elements that are depleted.

Your intention is also that if there is too much Chi in an element, the energy will put your body in a space where it can dissipate the energy, and will not exacerbate the imbalance.

Your intention is that the energies will bring into balance all the various correspondences of each element, not just the physical organs, which are just a small part of what each element represents.

So, as before, there are three intentions here: (1) boost depleted elements, (2) allow 'excess' elements to dissipate their excess, and (3) balance physical, mental, emotional and spiritual aspects of each element.

Wood

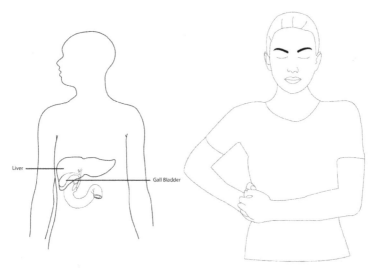

1. In whatever way feels right for you, imagine the source of the Reiki energy in the air above you. Connect to that energy.
2. Rest your hands on the Liver/Gall Bladder area, to the right side of your abdomen on the lower part of your ribcage. Rest one hand over the other.
3. Imagine cascades of energy/light flooding down into your crown, passing through your shoulders and arms, and flooding into your Liver and Gall Bladder.
4. Alternatively, maintain your focus on your Liver and Gall Bladder and allow the energy to flow there, without any active visualisation.

5. The energy keeps on flowing, continually renewed.
6. Maintain this focus for several minutes.

Fire

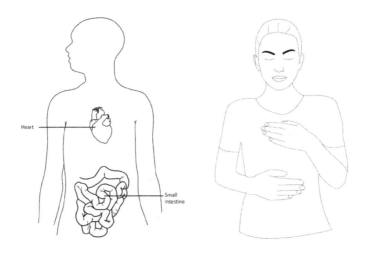

1. Rest your hands on the Heart and the Small Intestine, by placing your left hand to the left side of the midline of your chest (heart) and the right hand between the navel and the solar plexus.
2. Imagine cascades of energy/light flooding down into your crown, passing through your shoulders and arms, and flooding into your Heart and Small Intestine.

3. Have in mind the Triple Heater and the Heart Protector too.
4. Alternatively, maintain your focus on those organs and allow the energy to flow there, without any active visualisation.
5. The energy keeps on flowing, continually renewed.
6. Maintain this focus for several minutes.

Earth

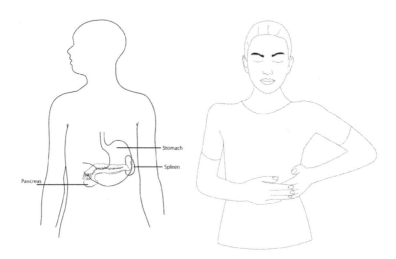

1. Rest your hands on the Spleen/Pancreas and Stomach area, by partly overlapping your hands as they rest on the stomach (left side of upper

abdomen) and spleen (left side of your abdomen on the lower part of your ribcage.

2. Imagine cascades of energy/light flooding down into your crown, passing through your shoulders and arms, and flooding into your Spleen/Pancreas and Stomach.

3. Alternatively, maintain your focus on those organs and allow the energy to flow there, without any active visualisation.

4. The energy keeps on flowing, continually renewed.

5. Maintain this focus for several minutes.

Metal

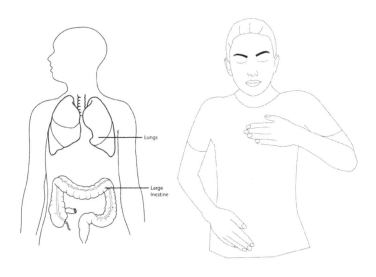

1. Rest your hands on the Lungs and Large Intestine: place one hand on the lung area on one side of the body, and the other hand on the other side of the body, on the lower abdomen. Half way through this self-treatment, swap hands, so you treat the other lung and the other side of the large intestine. Have in mind that when you are treating one lung, the energy will also be connecting with the other lung, and when you are treating the large intestine, have in mind that you will be connecting with the whole organ (ascending, transverse and descending colon).
2. Imagine cascades of energy/light flooding down into your crown, passing through your shoulders and arms, and flooding into your Lungs and Large Intestine.
3. Alternatively, maintain your focus on those organs and allow the energy to flow there, without any active visualisation.
4. The energy keeps on flowing, continually renewed.
5. Maintain this focus for several minutes.

Water

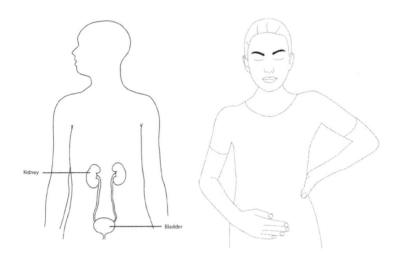

1. Rest your hands on the Kidneys and Bladder: Place one hand on the kidney on one side of the body, on your lower back where the ribcage stops, next to your spine; the other hand rests on your bladder in the midline of your lower abdomen. Half way through this self-treatment, swap hands, so you treat the other kidney, and the bladder again. When you are treating each individual kidney, have in mind that the energy will also be connecting with the other kidney.
2. Imagine cascades of energy/light flooding down into your crown, passing through your shoulders and arms, and flooding into your Kidneys and Bladder.

3. Alternatively, maintain your focus on those organs and allow the energy to flow there, without any active visualisation.
4. The energy keeps on flowing, continually renewed.
5. Maintain this focus for several minutes.

Move your hands back into your lap, palms uppermost, and spend a few minutes just experiencing the balance that ensues.

Or, if you were self-treating while lying down, just bring your hands together, folded over the heart area, and experience that sense of balance for a while.

Gentle 'Hands Off' Self-Treatment method

For this gentle hands-on self-treatment method, you can either sit on a chair or lie down on a treatment table. Close your eyes and take a couple of long deep breaths to settle yourself. Say to yourself "I am now going to bring my elements into balance".

As before, there are three intentions here: (1) boost depleted elements, (2) allow 'excess' elements to dissipate their excess, and (3) balance physical, mental, emotional and spiritual aspects of each element.

We start with Wood. You are familiar with the location of the corresponding 'organs' – Liver and Gall Bladder – so you can just let your attention rest there in your body. The energy will follow your focus and focus itself where your attention rests.

If you like, you can imagine that there are some hands resting on your body in that area, rather like when you were carrying out the hands-on self-treatment. This is optional but may be something that you might like to do.

Experiment and find out what works best for you.

Now move through the other elements in the order Fire, Earth, Metal and Water, each time focusing your attention on those 'organs' or imagining hands resting on them, and allow the energy to flow.

When you have finished, just spend a few minutes just experiencing the balance that ensues.

The Reiki "inner smile" meditation

If you are looking for a guided meditation to help you with this, I have framed this sort of self-treatment meditation as a Reiki "inner smile" meditation, where I talk you through focusing a sense of loving kindness towards your 'organs' and other aspects of each element.

Of course, as you do this, Reiki follows your focus and gently envelops and cradles each element.

You can find the meditation in the "MP3" section of my web site: www.reiki-evolution.co.uk

"Stronger" self-treatments

So, we're going to bring out the big guns now, by carrying out self-treatments that are more potent and penetrate more deeply. Here are the differences in what you are going to be doing, compared with what I have described before:

(1)   You'll definitely need to know what the state of your elements is before you start.
(2)   You are going to 'stabilise' your elements before you begin. This is something new!
(3)   You are going to use the Five Element symbols to generate the five energies at which your 'organs' resonate.
(4)   You will keep track of the state of each element as you treat it, using your intuition, so you know when to move on to the next element.

How long to spend on each element?

Earlier I suggested that you spend a few minutes on each element and that, if you knew the state of your elements when you began your treatment, you could spend more time working on the elements that were most out of balance.

This time you are going to use your intuition to keep track of what is happening with an element *as you treat it* so you know when you have built up an element that was deficient, or have dissipated energy from an element that held too much chi.

Once that happens, you can move on to the next element. So you stop treating an element when it has moved from, say, +25%, or -40%, to zero (balance).

What intuitive method to use

Use a method that does not involve stopping to open your eyes and grab a pendulum or use physical hand movements. Use a method that you can feel comfortable with, that allows you to know the state of an element, in your head, as you treat.

So whether you use imagined text, or an imaginary pendulum with protractor, or a slider or a mixing desk, or have a general impression of the state of an element... whatever works for you and is quick and easy: use that!

So in these 'stronger' self-treatments you will:

1. Find out what's happening with your elements
2. Use a symbol to stabilise them (see below)
3. Treat the elements with hands-on or visualisation
4. Notice the energy changes as you treat
5. Keep on going until they are balanced

How to 'stabilise' your elements before you start

This is a new stage, and it is a necessary one.

I have a new symbol for you that you can use to 'get the elements moving', awaken them, loosen them up, bring them into the sort of state that means they get the most out of the treatment you are going to give.

Interestingly, symbols that you can use with Reiki, to focus and direct energy, seem to fall into two categories:

1. Symbols that produce energy of a particular frequency
2. Symbols that produce a particular effect.

So SHK produces a high frequency energy that focuses on thoughts and emotions – 'heavenly ki', while the 'fire serpent' symbol (taught on the Reiki Evolution Master Teacher course) balances the chakras.

This symbol falls into the latter category: it produces balance. It balances the chakras, but it also benefits the elements, to prepare them and get them ready for change.

To use the symbol, draw the symbol out using your fingers – or visualise it being drawn out in your mind's eye – in front of you and imagine the symbol merging with your body, running from the crown of your head to the base of your spine.

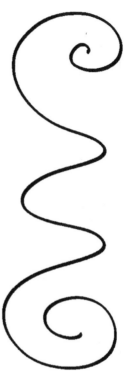

If you like, you can draw the symbol out in your mind's eye, without using your hands.

This symbol does not have a name that has to be repeated like a mantra.

Here is the symbol. Draw it from the top to the bottom…

Once you've done this, your elements are all ready for what comes next: the self-treatment proper.

Stronger 'Hands On' Self-Treatment method

So, you've intuited the state of your elements in some way and written it down, so you know which elements hold too much chi and which are deficient. Because of this, you also know which elements you'll probably be spending the most time working on, since the elements that are most out of balance take longer to bring into balance!

You've used the 'stabilising' symbol so that your elements are all ready, loosened up, open and expectant.

This hands-on self-treatment method can be carried out either while you're sitting in a chair of lying on a treatment couch.

If sitting, you can begin with your eyes closed and your hands resting in your lap, palms uppermost. If lying down, you can begin by resting your hands, folded, over your heart.

Say to yourself "I am now going to bring my elements into balance".

As before, your intention is threefold: (1) to boost depleted elements, (2) to allow 'excess' elements to dissipate their excess, and (3) to balance physical, mental, emotional and spiritual aspects of each element.

Wood

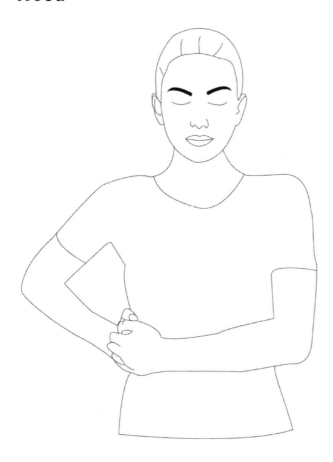

1. In your mind's eye, draw out the Wood symbol in the air above you, representing the source of that energy.
2. Rest your hands on the Liver/Gall Bladder area, to the right side of your abdomen on the lower part of your ribcage. Rest one hand over the other.
3. Imagine cascades of energy/light flooding down from that symbol into your crown, passing through your shoulders and arms, and flooding into your Liver and Gall Bladder.
4. Alternatively, maintain your focus on your Liver and Gall Bladder, have in mind that the energy is flowing there from that symbol and allow the energy to flow there, without any active visualisation.
5. The energy keeps on flowing, continually renewed.
6. Keep an eye on (intuit the state of) this element as you self-treat, and when the element is in balance, you can move on to the next element.

Fire

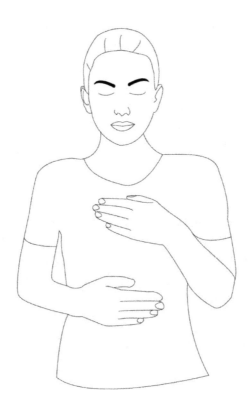

1. In your mind's eye, draw out the Fire symbol in the air above you, representing the source of that energy.
2. Rest your hands on the Heart and the Small Intestine, by placing your left hand to the left side of the midline of your chest (heart) and the right hand between the navel and the solar plexus.
3. Imagine cascades of energy/light flooding down from that symbol into your crown, passing through your shoulders and arms, and flooding into your Heart and Small Intestine.
4. Have in mind the Triple Heater and the Heart Protector too.
5. Alternatively, maintain your focus on those organs, have in mind that the energy is flowing there from that symbol and allow the energy to flow there, without any active visualisation.
6. The energy keeps on flowing, continually renewed.
7. Keep an eye on (intuit the state of) this element as you self-treat, and when the element is in balance, you can move on to the next element.

Earth

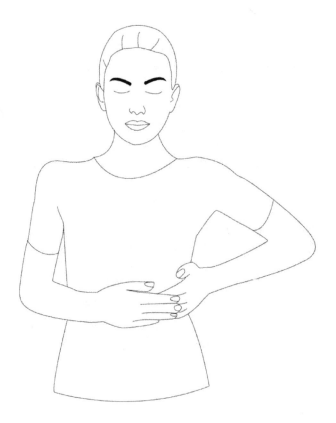

1. In your mind's eye, draw out the Earth symbol in the air above you, representing the source of that energy.
2. Rest your hands on the Spleen/Pancreas and Stomach area, by partly overlapping your hands as they rest on the stomach (left side of upper abdomen) and spleen (left side of your abdomen on the lower part of your ribcage.
3. Imagine cascades of energy/light flooding down from that symbol into your crown, passing through your shoulders and arms, and flooding into your Spleen/Pancreas and Stomach.
4. Alternatively, maintain your focus on those organs, have in mind that the energy is flowing there from that symbol and allow the energy to flow there, without any active visualisation.
5. The energy keeps on flowing, continually renewed.
6. Keep an eye on (intuit the state of) this element as you self-treat, and when the element is in balance, you can move on to the next element.

Metal

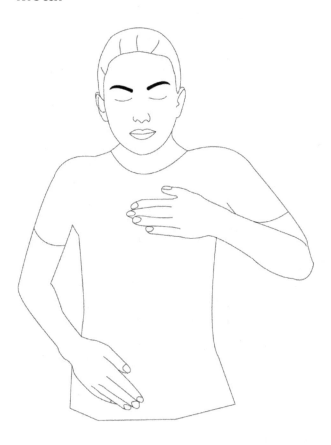

1. In your mind's eye, draw out the Metal symbol in the air above you, representing the source of that energy.
2. Rest your hands on the Lungs and Large Intestine: place one hand on the lung area on one side of the body, and the other hand on the other side of the body, on the lower abdomen. Half way through this self-treatment, swap hands, so you treat the other lung and the other side of the large intestine. Have in mind that when you are treating one lung, the energy will also be connecting with the other lung, and when you are treating the large intestine, have in mind that you will be connecting with the whole organ (ascending, transverse and descending colon).
3. Imagine cascades of energy/light flooding down from that symbol into your crown, passing through your shoulders and arms, and flooding into your Lungs and Large Intestine.
4. Alternatively, maintain your focus on those organs, have in mind that the energy is flowing there from that symbol and allow the energy to flow there, without any active visualisation.
5. The energy keeps on flowing, continually renewed.
6. Keep an eye on (intuit the state of) this element as you self-treat, and when the element is in balance, you can move on to the next element.

Water

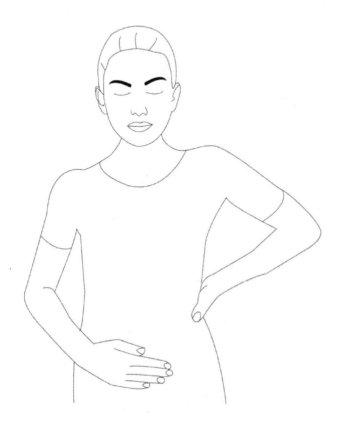

1. In your mind's eye, draw out the Water symbol in the air above you, representing the source of that energy.
2. Rest your hands on the Kidneys and Bladder: Place one hand on the kidney on one side of the body, on your lower back where the ribcage stops, next to your spine; the other hand rests on your bladder in the midline of your lower abdomen. Half way through this self-treatment, swap hands, so you treat the other kidney, and the bladder again. When you are treating each individual kidney, have in mind that the energy will also be connecting with the other kidney.
3. Imagine cascades of energy/light flooding down from that symbol into your crown, passing through your shoulders and arms, and flooding into your Kidneys and Bladder.
4. Alternatively, maintain your focus on those organsr, have in mind that the energy is flowing there from that symbol and allow the energy to flow there, without any active visualisation.
5. The energy keeps on flowing, continually renewed.
6. Keep an eye on (intuit the state of) this element as you self-treat, and when the element is in balance, you can bring this self-treatment to a close.

Move your hands back into your lap, palms uppermost, and spend a few minutes just experiencing the balance that ensues.

Or, if you are self-treating while lying down, just bring your hands together, folded over the heart area, and experience that sense of balance for a while.

Stronger 'Hands Off' Self-Treatment method

So, you've intuited the state of your elements in some way and written it down, so you know which elements hold too much chi and which are deficient. Because of this, you also know which elements you'll probably be spending the most time working on, since the elements that are most out of balance take longer to bring into balance!

You've used the 'stabilising' symbol so that your elements are all ready, loosened up, open and expectant.

This hands-off self-treatment method can be carried out either while you're sitting in a chair of lying on a treatment couch.

If sitting, you can begin with your eyes closed and your hands resting in your lap, palms uppermost. If lying down, you can begin by resting your hands, folded, over your heart or, if more comfortable, lying by your sides.

Say to yourself "I am now going to bring my elements into balance".

As before, your intention is threefold: (1) to boost depleted elements, (2) to allow 'excess' elements to dissipate their excess, and (3) to balance physical, mental, emotional and spiritual aspects of each element.

We start with Wood. Follow this sequence:

1. In your mind's eye, draw out the Wood symbol in the air above you, representing the source of that energy.

2. You are familiar with the location of the corresponding 'organs' – Liver and Gall Bladder – so you can let your attention rest there. Imagine cascades of energy/light flooding down from that symbol into your Liver and Gall Bladder.

3. Alternatively, maintain your focus on your Liver and Gall Bladder, have in mind that the energy is flowing there from that symbol and allow the energy to flow there, without any active visualisation.

4. If you like, you can imagine that there are some hands resting on your body in that area, rather like when you were carrying out the hands-on self-treatment. Energy floods into the Liver and Gall Bladder from that symbol.

5. The energy keeps on flowing, continually renewed.

6. Keep an eye on (intuit the state of) this element as you self-treat, and when the element is in balance, you can move on to the next element.

Now move through the other elements in the order Fire, Earth, Metal and Water, each time using the corresponding symbol, focusing your attention on those 'organs' or imagining hands resting on them, and allow the energy to flow until you have intuited that the element is balanced.

When you have finished, just spend a few minutes just experiencing the balance that ensues.

Self-Treatment Case History

Below you can see some bar charts representing the state of an individual's elements during a daily programme of 'hands-on' self-treatments, lasting 15 minutes at each session.

There is one bar chart for each element, showing how the state of that element changed from one session to another.

The first 'reading' – the reading for "Day 1" - shows the state of that element before the daily self-treatments began.

Let's start, though, with a snapshot of the person's five elements before they carried out any self-treatments:

State of Elements
Before Self-Treatments Started

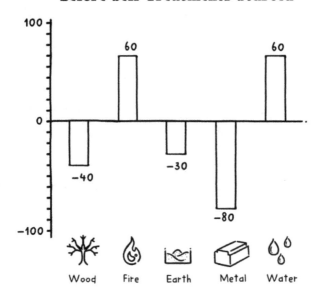

This is what happened to each of their elements during their daily self-treatments:

Wood:
Changes Over a 14 Day Period

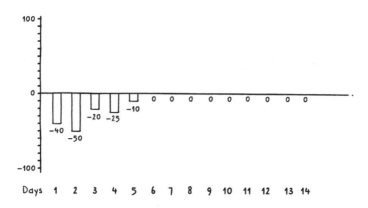

Fire:
Changes Over a 14 Day Period

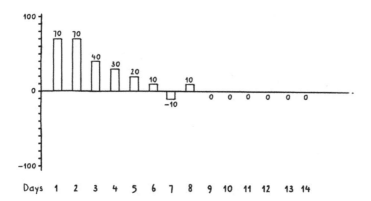

Earth:
Changes Over a 14 Day Period

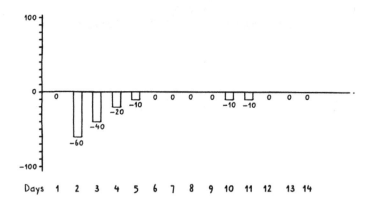

Metal:
Changes Over a 14 Day Period

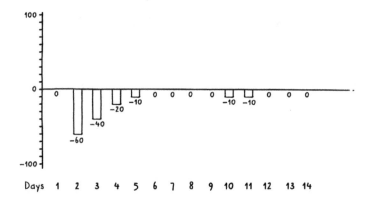

Water:
Changes Over a 14 Day Period

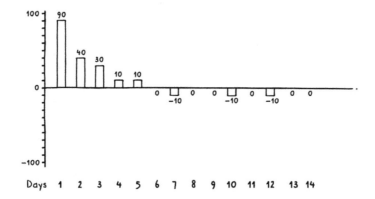

Working on Other People

Introduction

When you work on other people using the Five Element Reiki system, you will follow the same sort of stages that you have already used when working on yourself, so a lot of this will already be familiar to you.

Stage 1: Intuit the imbalances

The first stage of Five Element treatments is to find out where the imbalances are.

You can use whatever intuitive approach you feel comfortable with but it will be a lot easier for you if you can intuit 'in your head' rather than using some sort of a physical prop.

As before, each element will hold too much chi, too little chi, or will be in balance.

If you like, you can intuit the state of your client's elements before they arrive for their appointment. By doing it that way, your intuition will not be affected at all by what they tell you when they arrive for their appointment... if you were concerned that your intuition might be affected in that way.

Stage 2: stabilise and prepare the elements

Once you have intuited the state of the elements (and written that down somewhere!), you then move on to stabilise and prepare the elements. This needs to be done before the treatment proper can begin, and you already know what symbol you can use to achieve this.

Stage 3: treat the elements

Finally, here comes the 'treatment proper': you can use five element energies to 'flush through' each element's 'organs' and meridians, whereupon the energies will focus on bringing into balance all the various correspondences of that element in our body-mind-spirit.

You will spend comparatively more time flushing through the elements that were most out of balance, though you will spend some time on each of them, just to 'touch base' and get things moving in all elements and on all levels, empowering all of the elements to support and restrain each other to achieve balance.

You will keep an eye on the state of the elements, intuitively, as you go through the treatment, so you know when to move on from one element to another.

Perceiving Someone Else's Elements

There are several ways of finding out whether there are any imbalances in someone's elements.

Many of them have already been described in the section "Monitoring the state of one's elements" and it would be a good idea if you went back to that section to re-familiarise yourself with its contents.

You will have read about:

1. Receiving general impressions
2. Dowsing using a pendulum
3. Imaginary pendulums
4. Using imagined text
5. Using sliders
6. The 'mixing desk'
7. Using physical hand-movements

You have already been practising intuiting the state of your own elements and you can use those same approaches to intuit the state of someone else's.

Perhaps you have already settled on your most comfortable method, and if so then you will probably do well using that method for other people too.

When you are treating yourself, it is useful to be able to sense the state of the elements using an 'in your head' method, so that you can monitor what is going on with an element while you treat it.

This is just as useful a skill when you are treating other people.

Nevertheless, in this section I am introducing a new method that you might think about using, or experimenting with. This method comes under the heading of "Hara diagnosis" and involves sensing energy above the recipient's Hara, and is a form of 'scanning'.

There is a way of doing this that involves pressing different areas of the the Hara but prodding someone's abdomen with your fingertips is a very non-Reiki thing to do, it has to be said, so I'm not including that here! Sensing over that Hara is more Reiki-like!

You may choose not to investigate this method, and that's fine.

Ultimately you are likely to end up relying on intuitive diagnosis rather than scanning, since this is the most effortless approach.

A Window On The Elements

Hara diagnosis, which is used in Shiatsu, offers you a 'window' that you can look through, metaphorically, to peer in at the condition of the elements.

Too much looking can cause the picture to change, though, so when sensing imbalances in this way you need to learn to be fairly speedy and confident and decisive.

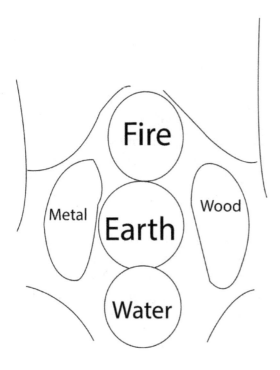

Sensing Over the Hara

You can see from the diagram above that different areas of the abdomen represent each element. By scanning over these areas, you can detect imbalances.

It can take some practice before you feel completely confident with this technique, so you may need to persevere.

You hover one hand over the Hara, focusing your attention on the sensations in your palm/fingers, checking the areas corresponding to each element, each time comparing one element with another.

By feeling the quality of the energies you can gauge whether there is too much Chi (jitsu) or too little Chi (kyo) in each element, and you can use this approach to back up what you concluded when you were intuiting the state of your client's elements.

This approach only really lets you find the elements with the greatest excess and the greatest deficiency of Chi, and cannot normally be used to discern more subtle gradations of imbalance, unless you are particularly sensitive to the energy.

You are already used to experiencing and feeling energy in your hands, of course, so you are better sensitised to begin with than people on Shiatsu courses who are learning this method and who have not been attuned to Reiki!

Intention

Firstly, set your intention so that you are going to feel energetic imbalances in the five elements in the Hara area.

Your intention is important here: you will not be picking up physical problems in the body below you, and you will not be picking up things in the chakras. Your intent is focused on diagnosing five element imbalances in the Hara.

Don't try too hard

When you are practicing this stage it is important that you don't try too hard. Just play around with the method, simply see what you notice, and go on your first impressions.

If you try too hard you can almost put a block in the way, so relax and be neutral. Simply notice in a detached way what happens.

The experience of one of our students illustrates this point:

"I have spent the last few months practising detecting imbalances on my clients. I have been doing the tests both before and after my normal Reiki sessions. Initially I could sense nothing, but once I stopped trying to force a response and "let it happen", I started to get results."

What will I feel?

When the elements are in balance you can feel a uniform energy, rather like riding on a carpet. As you are scanning, feel for empty holes within the 'carpet' layer, and feel for differences between the different elements/areas.

A 'hole' or a feeling of dullness or emptiness would indicate that there is insufficient Chi in that area; maybe you would feel coldness there.

If you feel heat, or some sort of bright fizzing or tingling or pulsing, or an up-draught of wind perhaps, then there is likely to be an excess of Chi in that element.

Scanning

Here is a suggested routine:

1. Start by comparing, say, Fire and Earth; feel one, then the other, and maybe quickly drift from

one to the other and back again. Which is kyo and which is jitsu?

2. Now move on to another element, say Metal. If Metal feels kyo, then compare it with the element that felt kyo last time: which is the most kyo... remember that element as the most deficient. If Metal feels jitsu, then compare it with the element that felt jitsu last time: which is the most jitsu... remember that element as the one with the greatest excess of chi.

3. Now move on to another element, say Wood. If it is kyo, then compare its quality with the most kyo element that you have found so far, and decide which element is now the most kyo that you have yet come across. If Wood is jitsu, then compare its quality with the most jitsu element that you have found so far, and decide which element is now the most jitsu that you have yet come across.

4. Now move on to the remaining element, which in this case is Water. Again compare its quality of kyo or jitsu with the most jitsu and most kyo elements that you have found so far.

5. By Comparing one element with another and moving on, you can thus decide which element has the greatest excess of chi, and which element is most deficient.

When carrying out this process you need to go on your first impression, and try not to analyse things too much.

If you keep on moving back and forth, back and forth, you will 'lose it' completely, it will all feel like porridge and your intervention will start to alter the Hara presentation. So you need to decide quickly.

Don't dither: just decide and move on.

With practice, you won't need to be so deliberate and methodical with your movements and comparisons: you will be able to drift your hand around quite quickly, in a very fluid and flowing fashion, noticing the most full (jitsu) and the most empty (kyo) elements.

If you can detect more subtle differences, that would enable you to put all five elements in order from jitsu to kyo, on the basis of scanning alone, you warrant congratulations for being so sensitive to the energy!

Making sense of the imbalances you find

Quite often the imbalances 'fit' with the control and nourishment cycles, so for example when Metal is up, Wood is down, because Metal controls Wood etc... but the imbalances you detect will not always be so neat and tidy!

The way the elements interact can be quite complicated and difficult to fathom, but that's fine because you don't have to work it all out: all we do is simply accept the state of the elements and take action based on what we find. So don't blow your mind trying to understand 'why': simply accept what you find and move on.

It is interesting to see how a person's imbalances tie in with what you know of their physical, mental and emotional state, and the correspondences of the elements.

Many times what you find will 'make sense' but don't worry too much if it doesn't always make sense.

Here are some students' experiences of imbalances that made sense in terms of the correspondences of the elements...

"One interesting example was a friend of mine who when stressed develops a stutter and I found that the Fire element was very depleted. The next time I saw them to practice on, they happened to mention that they had had a very anxiety making moment and had managed not to stutter nearly as much and had found a clarity rather than a panic when they started stuttering. I hadn't mentioned to them anything about stuttering and had only been aware of it after the treatment and I had gone to re-read my course notes."

"One lady I treated in her home who suffers liver cancer. On the first treatment I did "just" Reiki. Second visit she started to open up more about her life and her hate/anger/bitterness of her mother. I scanned for 5E, knowing of course of the liver cancer, and decided to remove some of the excess energy from the liver and to balance things up. But the more energy I removed the more the hatred poured out. I approached the idea of letting go and forgiveness etc but she was adamant that she would hate her mother until the day she died. On the third treatment she was very, very ill, she complained bitterly that the pain relief was not working and that she didn't deserve to suffer this pain, that the doctors should sort out her medication better. She was on chemo tablets and she shouldn't need to have the pain as well. Her eyes were pure yellow and I was shocked by the anger and bitterness that seemed to spew from her."

Some examples

I started a series of treatments on J.

When I hovered my hand over the Hara, Fire seemed to be the most 'dull' or 'empty' - there seemed to be a 'hole' in the Hara 'carpet' in that area. When I hovered over Metal, it seemed to be the most bright, fierce, tense or strong.

Then I went on to use an intuitive technique, which gave the presentation shown below. It is displayed as a Bar Chart.

The numbers relating to 'excess' or 'depletion' are purely subjective, of course, but give an impression of the relative levels of excess or deficiency.

The order of the elements shown is Wood - Fire - Earth - Metal -Water. Water was in balance.

Let's try and make sense of this (we don't have to do this, but it's an interesting mental exercise in putting into practice some of the things that we know about the elements and how they support and control each other).

State of Five Elements for "J"

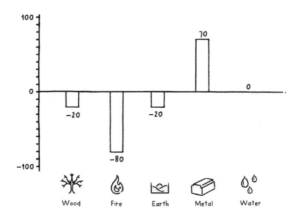

Fire was depleted, so it was not supporting Earth, which was also down a little. Fire controls Metal, but since Fire was so depleted, it could not control Metal, which raged uncontrolled.

Maybe Metal was so strong that it depleted its controlling element: Fire. Metal controls Wood, and Metal was very strong so Wood was suppressed.

These interpretations are just speculation really, but we can see in the above example how the different elements connect with each other, supporting or failing to support, controlling or failing to control.

Some Questions For You

In the previous example ("J"):

1.   What emotional states might this person be experiencing?
2.   What states of mind might they be exhibiting?
3.   What parts of the physical body might be affected in some way?

Example 1

Speculate about the relationship between the elements in this person.

1.   What emotional states might they be experiencing?
2.   What states of mind might they be exhibiting?
3.   What parts of the physical body might be affected in some way?

EXAMPLE 1

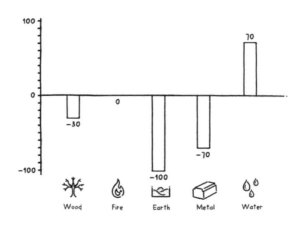

Example 2

Speculate about the relationship between the elements in this person.

1.   What emotional states might they be experiencing?
2.   What states of mind might they be exhibiting?
3.   What parts of the physical body might be affected in some way?

EXAMPLE 2

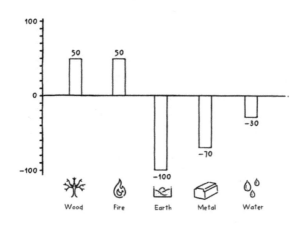

Student Comments About Hara Diagnosis

"I have been working with detecting energy imbalances and have found it quite amazing especially when the results became consistent... No problem with feeling the energies because for a couple of years now my hands vibrate naturally when detecting energy imbalances in treatments and distance healing using intent/scanning. Once I got this method under control it was possible to confirm with dowsing."
Jeannie, England

"I am now doing 5eH imbalance detection on all of my clients. Some of them show a strong imbalance others less or minimal. I've noticed that the clients showing a strong imbalance tend to be those who have come with a specific ailment that they want me to concentrate on. Those who have just come for relaxation tend to be less strong in their imbalance."
John, Wales

"I did a balancing on Caron yesterday (she did Reiki years ago and practices reflexology now) she was the most 'balanced' person I've had yet, from a 'starting point' of view. She was Wood -10; Fire 0; Earth -10; Metal 0; Water +20. It is interesting to see that people who are more focused and 'spiritual' and practise

healing in some way or another tend to be more balanced than those that aren't. Obvious statement really, but is amazing to have it confirmed by their readings."
Ellen, England

"Another client said she felt as if I had given her a whole bodywork like a massage. She is going through emotional upset and having trouble with her eyes. Her Wood was 100% excess - never before had I associated anger with her but when we discussed it she admitted to having a lot of anger buried deep inside. She also had excessive Earth (20%) and excessive Water (60%). It all tied in with what is going on in her life."
Jeannie, England

"I am really excited! Have done another 'detecting' on a new 'guinea pig', Joanne, and understood a bit more as the Acupuncture - 5 elements book had come in. I am absolutely blown away (and so was she!) it's as if you can read the actual person like a book! I didn't really know anything about her before along these lines, but she confirmed so many things. It is incredible and I said to Paul 'this really works!' and there is also far more to it (far reaching) than I ever thought."
Ellen, England

"I've practised diagnosis on 11 people, most more than once. The results have been quite astonishing. I realised this when I began to practice on family and friends who had more serious problems than friends who didn't - with

healthy friends I was getting very minor imbalances, or a couple who were completely balanced. When I started to try it out on family with more problems (parents mainly!) results were much more obvious. This was a really good comparison and gave me a lot of confidence."
Maurita, England

Stabilising and Preparing Someone's Elements

The 'stabilising' symbol

You were introduced to this symbol in the 'Self-treatments' section, so you know about it already: it is used to 'get the elements moving', awaken them, loosen them up, bring them into the sort of state that means they get the most out of the treatment you are going to give.

The symbol prepares the elements and get them ready for change.

To use the symbol, draw the symbol out using your fingers – or visualise it being drawn out in your mind's eye along the length of the recipient, running from the crown of their head to the base of their spine.

If you like, you can draw the symbol out in your mind's eye, without using your hands. This symbol does not have a name that has to be repeated like a mantra. Once you've done this, your client is ready for what comes next: the treatment proper.

Treating the Elements

Introduction

Our treatment approach derives from the Japanese traditions of te-ate ('hand application') or tanasue-no-michi ('the Tao of placing hands'), which have been known for centuries, and are described in the book 'Macrobiotic Palm Healing' by Michio Kushi (see Reading List).

Teate is a way of balancing a person's energy system, and is based on knowledge of the chakras, the meridian system and the five elements.

The system does not involve attunements, but many of the approaches echo techniques used in Reiki, and some of Mikao Usui's surviving students referred to his system as 'Usui Teate'.

Working on organ pairs

While Teate can be used to direct healing energy into a single organ, there are benefits in working on pairs of organs, the organs that represent each element.

The organs that represent an element are balanced in terms of Yin and Yang: one organ has a Yang structure and Yin energy, the other has a Yin structure and Yang energy.

The organs are associated and complementary: one influences the other and they share a closely co-ordinated energy flow.

So, for example, by working simultaneously on the Lungs and the Large Intestine (the organs/meridians of Metal) we produce a stronger healing effect than if we worked on the individual organs separately, and in Five Element Reiki we intensify the healing effect further by using energies that resonate at the characteristic frequencies of the organs.

What I am going to do in this section is to outline three different treatment approaches that you can use, and you should experiment with them to see what's possible and what you get on well with. We start with a very simple hands-on method where you rest your hands on the recipient's body in five set positions, connect to the corresponding symbol and let the energy do what it needs to do.

Then, I'll describe a more intense or potent hands-on treatment method where you deliberately boost the chi in an element, or drain the chi from an element, keeping an eye on the element's state while you're treating.

Finally, we'll talk about a treatment method that you can carry out entirely in your head, using intent and visualisation, without using any hand positions: without taking your hands off your client's shoulders at all.

Treatment Option 1: Treating the Elements Simply

This is the main part of the treatment, starting with 5-10 minutes resting our hands on the shoulders to get Reiki flowing and bringing the client into a nice relaxed state.

Procedure

What we are going to do then is to connect with the pairs of 'organs' that represent each element, send the corresponding five element energy through them, concentrating (spending more time) on the elements that were most out of balance.

We will take about 50 minutes to complete the sequence, giving a treatment lasting about an hour.

1. Place your hands on the corresponding 'organs'
2. Connect to the elemental energy by imagining the symbol in the air above you
3. Draw down energy from that symbol, through your crown, through your shoulders and hands, into the 'organs'

4. Now let the energy flow, drawing down energy as necessary, or just bliss out and let the energy flow as it wants
5. Continue until you get the impression that balance has been achieved

Your intention

You are going to be flooding each element with its corresponding energy and your intention needs to be that this energy will either boost the chi of elements that are deficient, or will support an element in dissipating its excess chi.

You don't want to 'pump' more chi into an already over-full element, so your intention is important here: the energy will support and allow the release of excess chi.

Please note also that when you use the energies in this way, your intention is that the energies will help your own energies to move more into a state of balance, releasing or building the chi in different elements, as necessary to achieve balance for you.

Timing

On a first visit, you will be guided by the presentation of the elements that you diagnose. If you have intuited the two elements that are most out of balance, spend more time working on those elements.

If you were able to intuit more detailed information about the degree of imbalance of each element, then you could 'grade' accordingly the amount of time that you spend working on each one.

Or you can just be guided by what happens to the state of the elements as you treat them: intuit their state to keep track of what's happening during the treatment, and when an element is balanced, move on to the next one.

Alternatively, you can also let your hands tell you when it is time to move on: if the energy is flowing intensely into one element, stay there until the sensations subside (within reason) or until you feel that it is right to move on now.

Do not leave out any of the elements: even if an element seems to be in balance, spend some time allowing the energy to flow there, stirring things up and allowing one element to influence another. You are, in effect, 'empowering' all the elements to support and restrain other elements, to achieve balance.

Element 'movements'

On subsequent visits, particularly if you are aware of the finer gradations of imbalance, the 'movement' of the elements can guide you as well.

If an element has swung strongly from being in excess to being deficient, or vice versa, then you might decide to spend more time on it irrespective of whether it displays the greatest excess or greatest deficiency.

So If Earth, say, had swung from +80 to -10 in one week, make sure that you spend a fair amount of time working on Earth even though it's only showing a small imbalance now: it has shifted a lot and still needs support.

Also think about the case of an element that is found to be in balance, or near balance, but was greatly out of balance in previous sessions. It has improved a lot over recent weeks, and you might decide to spend more time on that element than the 'snapshot' of the elements on that occasion might suggest is necessary, in order to 'reinforce' or 'lock in' the substantial change/movement that you have seen.

Step 1

Channel wood energy into the liver and gall bladder.

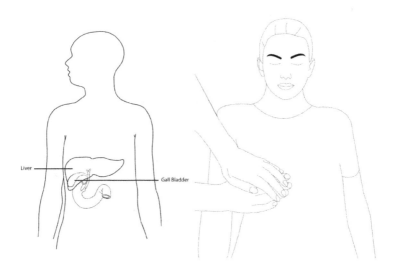

Rest both hands, overlapping each other, over the liver area. This is on the right side of the recipient's upper abdomen, wrapping round the side of the torso, where the rib cage stops.

Step 2

Channel fire energy into the heart and small intestine.

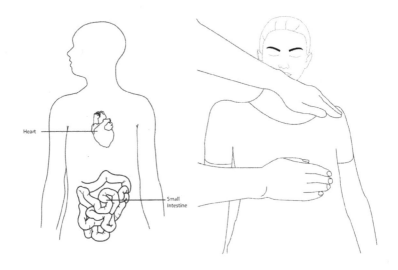

Rest one hand over the anatomical heart (or hover your hand in the case of a lady).
Rest the other hand on the abdomen, between the navel and the solar plexus.

Step 3

Channel earth energy into the stomach and spleen/pancreas.

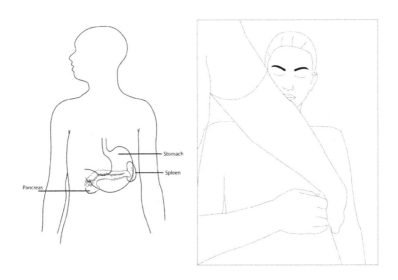

Rest both hands, slightly overlapping each other, on the upper abdomen. Stomach is to the left side of the recipient's upper abdomen. Spleen is on the left side of the recipient's torso, where the rib cage stops.

Step 4

Channel metal energy into the lungs and large intestine.

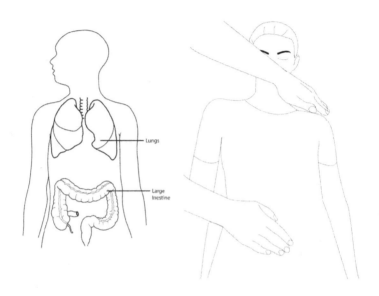

Rest one hand on one side of the lower abdomen, and the other hand hovers over (or rests on) the opposite lung. Intend that you are connecting with both lungs, and the entire large Intestine. Now swap over, and deal with the other side of the large intestine and other lung.

Step 5

Channel water energy into the kidney and bladder.

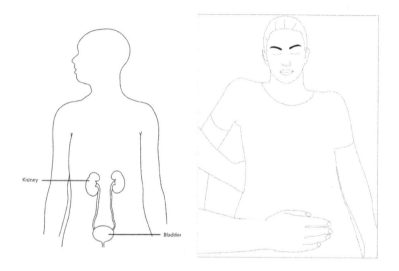

Rest one hand on the centre of the lower abdomen.
Slide the other hand slightly underneath the lower back,
where the ribcage stops. Intend that you are connecting
with the other kidney at the same time. Alternatively,
swap over half way and contact the other kidney, and
the bladder.

Step 6

Finishing the treatment

Perhaps finish the treatment by resting your hands on the feet/ankles for a while, a nice way to bring things to a close.

Treating in the Seated position

While Reiki treatments tend to be carried out with the recipient lying on a treatment couch, Teate would have been carried out with the recipient sitting, most likely sitting in 'seiza'.

Such treatments would have given the practitioner access to both sides of the body at the same time, and there were seen to be added benefits in working on the front of one organ and the back of another.

This approach was said to produce a more 'polarised' energy flow, and maybe you might like to experiment with this, though seiza is often a very uncomfortable sitting position for many Westerners, so you might want to alter this aspect.

Option 2: Treating the Elements using Visualisation

This is the main part of the treatment, starting with 5-10 minutes resting our hands on the shoulders to get Reiki flowing and bringing the client into a nice relaxed state.

Procedure

What we are going to do then is to connect with the pairs of 'organs' that represent each element, send the corresponding five element energy through them, concentrating (spending more time) on the elements that were most out of balance.

We will take about 50 minutes to complete the sequence, giving a treatment lasting about an hour.

What s different from Option 1 is that we are going to be actively visualising, not just allowing the energy to do what needs to be done. So this treatment can be seen as more intense, more powerful, because we are focusing the energy on working in a particular way.

This is rather like the difference between a gentle 'standard' Reiki treatment, where you just let the energy flow, and one where you use a symbol or a kotodama to intensify the healing effect.

We will visualise in a different way, depending on whether an element holds to little chi or too much chi. You will either be boosting the chi in an element that holds too little, quite deliberately, or 'deflating' an element that holds too much chi.

If There Is Too Little Chi

If there is too little chi in an element then you do this:

1. Place your hands on the corresponding 'organs'. See the "Option 1" section (above) for images of the hand positions to use.
2. Connect to the elemental energy by imagining the symbol in the air above you
3. Draw down energy from that symbol, through your crown, through your shoulders and hands, into the 'organs'
4. Now let the energy flow, imagining that the energy is filling up, replenisihing and boosting the energy in this element
5. Keep an eye on the state of the element intuitively and continue until you get the impression that balance has been achieved; then you can move on.

If There Is Too Much Chi

If there is too much chi in an element then you do this:

1. Place your hands on the corresponding 'organs'.
2. Connect to the elemental energy by imagining the symbol in the air above you
3. Using hand-movements, or intent, withdraw chi from the element/'organs'. Pull energy out of the organs and throw it away from you, pull out imaginary strands of excess energy, imagine that the organs are gently and powerfully allowing excess chi to escape like air, or vapour, rather like a relaxing exhalation that eliminates all tightness or denseness and brings everything down to the right relaxed level.
4. Keep an eye on the state of the element intuitively and continue until you get the impression that balance has been achieved; then you can move on.

Finishing the treatment

Perhaps finish the treatment by resting your hands on the feet/ankles for a while, a nice way to bring things to a close.

Your Intention

Unlike Option 1, where you were allowing the energy to do what was needed to either boost or deplete an element's energy, here you are taking control yourself and deliberately boosting or draining an element's energy in quite an intense way. So you need to have the ability to monitor the state of the elements 'in your head' as you treat.

Please note also that when you use the energies in this way, your intention is that the energies will help your own energies to move more into a state of balance, releasing or building the chi in different elements, as necessary to achieve balance for you.

Timing

On a first visit, you will be guided by the presentation of the elements that you diagnose. You will have intuited detailed information about the degree of imbalance of each element.

You can be guided by what happens to the state of the elements as you treat them: intuit their state to keep track of what's happening during the treatment, and when an element is balanced you can move on to the next one.

Do not leave out any of the elements: even if an element seems to be in balance, spend some time just allowing the energy to flow there, with the intention that it will do whatever is necessary, by way of stirring things up and allowing one element to influence another.

You are, in effect, 'empowering' all the elements to support and restrain other elements, to achieve balance.

Your Intuition

It would be really cumbersome for you to have to keep on stopping during this treatment, to pick up a pendulum, for example, to find out what was happening to the state of an element as you treated it. That would be so disrupting for your client and for you.

So you need to be comfortable with using some sort of 'in your head' method to perceive what is happening with an element 'on the fly'.

You should have experimented during the 'Self treatments' section and discovered what works best for you, so whether you get on best with an imaginary pendulum, an imaginary slider or a visualised mixing desk, or whether you find that you are most comfortable looking at text, hearing words or phrases, or just 'knowing' in some way what is happening with an element… use that method!

Option 3: Treating the Elements using Intent only (and not moving!)

This is an approach that you may or may not be interested in exploring, but I have included it to demonstrate how powerful the combination of intuition and intent can be.

What you are going to do is to carry out the entire treatment while sitting at the head of the treatment table, resting your hands on the client's shoulders.

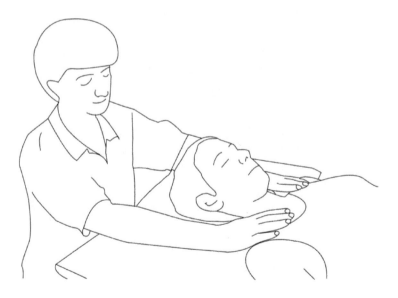

You do not change hand position.
You do not open your eyes.

You merge with the energy, use your intuition to determine the state of each element, and use intent to treat the elements and their associated 'organs'.

This is what to do...

Starting by spending 5-10 minutes resting your hands on the shoulders to get Reiki flowing and bringing the client into a nice relaxed state.

Working on Wood

Let's assume that there is a deficiency of chi in Wood. You have intuited this as you make contact with the element and its 'organs'.

Visualise the Wood symbol up in the air above you, representing the source of energy. Fix your attention of the approximate physical location of the Liver and Gall Bladder in the recipient's body. Be still. Imagine that energy is flooding down into those organs from the symbol above you; imagine that energy is flooding into you, through your arms, through your hands, into the recipient's body and on to their Liver and Gall Bladder.

You can either allow the energy to do whatever needs to be done to boost the chi in this element, or you can actively visualize boosting, filling and replenishing that element.

Every once in a while intuit the state of Wood, in your head, to see whether it has been boosted into a position of balance. If it hasn't, keep on boosting. If it has, move on to the next element: Fire.

Working on Fire

Let's assume that Fire is in balance. You have intuited this as you make contact with the element and its 'organs'.

Imagine the Fire symbol up in the air above the body and visualise the energy coming down to 'touch' the Heart and Small Intestine, the Heart Protector and the Triple Heater.

Just connect the organs to the energies for a few moments, until it feels right to move on. Allow the energy to stir up Fire, get the energies moving, empowering Fire to best support and restrain other elements.

Now we move on to Earth.

Working on Earth

Let's say that Earth holds an excess of chi. You have intuited this as you make contact with the element and its 'organs'.

Visualise the Earth symbol up in the air above you, representing the source of energy. Fix your attention of the approximate physical location of the Spleen and Stomach in the recipient's body. Visualise the energy coming down to 'touch' the Spleen and Stomach. Be still.

You can either allow the energy to do whatever needs to be done to release that excess energy, or you can actively visualize, imagining the excess chi flooding or escaping, gently and powerfully, reducing the tightness or density, while still connected to the Earth symbol above.

Every once in a while intuit the state of Earth, in your head, to see whether it has been returned to a position of balance. If it hasn't, keep on working on it. If it has, move on to the next element: Metal.

Working on Metal and Water

Deal with Metal, and then deal with Water. They will be balanced, they will hold an excess of chi or they will show a deficiency. You know what to do with these three presentations and all this can be done while you are simply resting your hands on the recipient's shoulders.

Fluidity

I am trying to free you from the physical rituals, and to help you realise that you can guide the process by simply merging with the energy and using your intuition and intent in a wonderful 'still' state.

Rather like going with the flow when you're playing the piano, merging with the music, becoming the music... you are connected to something more than the physical movements of your fingers.

Or maybe like improvising a solo on the guitar: you and the sound and the movements are fluid, part of one flow. Or maybe like the feeling you have when you do distant healing: you are part of the flow; with Five Element Reiki you are nudging, testing, guiding, moulding, monitoring, in a lovely fluid dance.

Client expectations

I should add that you do need to think about what your client is expecting from the treatment, because having you sitting motionless at the head of the treatment table for an extended period of timemay not be what they were anticipating, and they might not be too happy with that, or might think that you weren't really doing anything if they are new to such treatments.

If the client has seen you on previous occasions and trusts you, and has experienced benefits from the work that you have done together, they are likely to be more receptive if you explain what you are planning to do.

The benefits of compassionate touch

Also, we need to remember that there is something very special about compassionate, human touch, whether mixed up with energy work or not, and your client may be missing out from the benefits of gentle hands-on human contact during the treatment if you do not use different hand positions.

It is for you to experiment and find a way of working that honours your client's expectations and fits with the way that feels most appropriate for you to work.

Mixing Five Element Treatments with standard Reiki

Although sometimes a Five Element treatment can take 50-60 minutes, that is not always the case and often you may find that you have time 'left over' when you have worked through the five elements.

This is an ideal opportunity to work intuitively, using the Japanese "Reiji ho" method taught on Reiki Evolution Second Degree courses, where you still your mind and allow the energy to guide your hands to the right places to treat.

Alternatively, you can start a standard Reiki treatment and while you are resting your hands on someone's shoulders at the start of the treatment, you could choose to look at their elemental imbalances and bring the elements into balance using intent, checking the elements' state of balance in real time, before moving on to continue the treatment using standard or (ideally) intuitively-guided hand positions.

Treatment Case Histories

Case History #1:

Emotional Release

I treated one of my Reiki2 students, who was not feeling too good, and who could feel discomfort in her throat to solar plexus when she did her daily Hatsu Rei ho.

When I treated her, she has an enormous emotional release near the end of the first treatment, and she felt emotional for the next five days, crying and weeping. The second treatment was a great deal more restrained and seemed to resolve the problem.

On the first visit, the throat, heart and solar plexus chakras were closed down, but the first two had opened nicely by the time of the second treatment.

When I looked at the elements, there was no energy in Metal, the emotion associated with which is grief. I asked the lady if her strong emotional reaction was tied in with losing someone or something and she said "It's funny you should say that, but the last week when I have been crying, it has felt like grief."

She could not work out what the grief could be to begin with, but then she realised that it concerned a cousin of hers who had died young, and the loss of a horse.

When she did Hatsu Rei ho in the following week, most of the discomfort had gone, leaving only a little discomfort in the solar plexus. After the second treatment, this disappeared, and a few days later I found that all her elements were in balance, and none of her chakras were closed down.

This was interesting for me because the information from the chakras and the elements indicated that there was emotional stuff to be dealt with, and that the emotion that needed to be dealt with primarily was grief.

The lady concerned has also trained in Five Element Reiki and added this:

"What I found particularly interesting is that I had been suffering from eczema on my shins, not something I'd had before - it was bad enough that they were bleeding. I had tried all the usual things - E45 cream, checking soaps and detergents I was using and changing them - and nothing was clearing it up. When the grief cleared so did the eczema and of course metal is associated with the skin. I use this as an example of the dangers of assumptions about physical conditions, how western thinking would never associate eczema on the shins with grief and yet clearly there was a connection."

Case History # 2

The Bar Charts below show the element imbalances for a person who had a series of treatments over consecutive weeks, and show how the imbalances changed - and improved - over time.

This person had some very longstanding and debilitating problems.

Case History #2:
Before Any Treatments Started

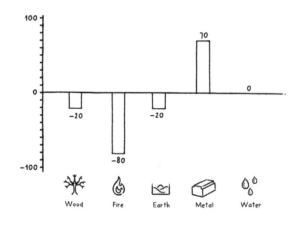

Case History #2: At The Second Visit

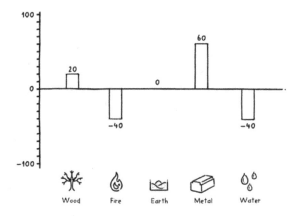

Case History #2: At The Third Visit

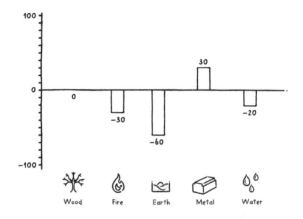

243

Case History #2: At The Fourth Visit

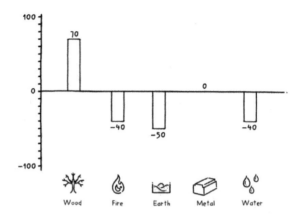

Case History #2: At The Fifth Visit

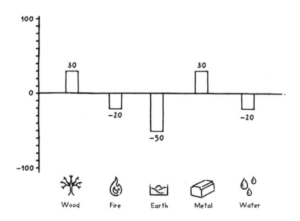

Case History #2: At The Sixth Visit

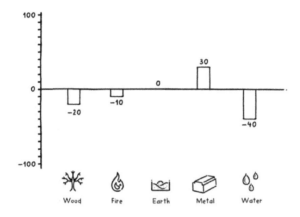

What is interesting here is that the beneficial changes produced by the course of treatments actually continued, and her elements came further into balance, during the three-week period following the end of the course of treatments.

Case History #2:
One Week After Treatments Ceased

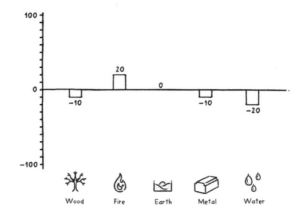

Case History #2:
Three Weeks After Treatments Ceased

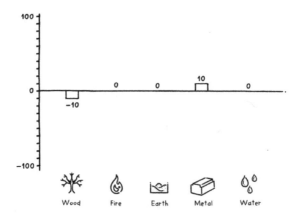

This shows that Five Element Reiki does not just produce short-term effects while you are actively treating a person, but continues to move the elements further into balance for some time after the final treatment. Here is the state of the elements at the start and end of the test period:

Comparison of the state of the elements at the start and end of the process

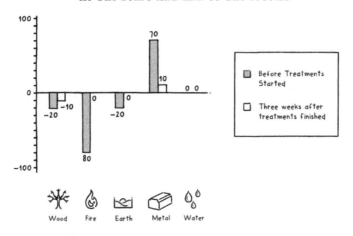

Comparison Of The State Of The Elements
At The Start And End Of The Process

Case History # 3

The Bar Charts below show the element imbalances for a person who had a few treatments over consecutive weeks, and show how the imbalances changed from one session to the next.

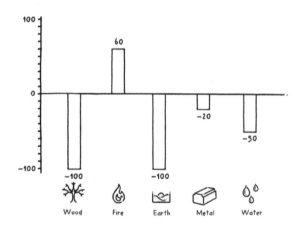

Case History #3:
Before Any Treatments Started

Case History #3:
At The Second Visit

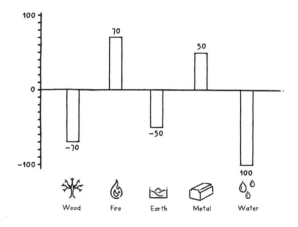

Case History #3:
At The Third Visit

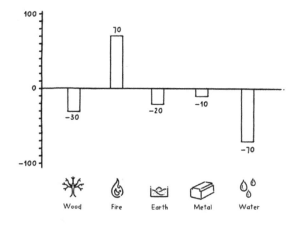

Case History #3:
At The Fourth Visit

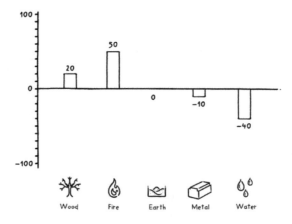

The course of treatments made a significant difference to the state of this person's elements, and you can see this better in the bar chart below where we compare the state of their elements before they had received any treatments with the state of their elements when they arrived for their fourth treatment.

Comparison of the state of the elements at the start and at visit 4

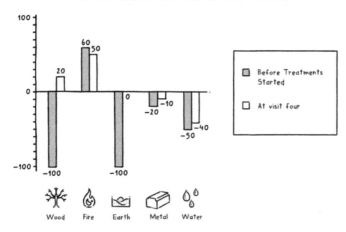

**Comparison Of The State Of The Elements
At The Start And End Of The Process**

You can see that the great deficiencies in Wood and Earth have completely disappeared and have been replaced by a balanced state. In addition, the excess in Fire, and the deficiencies in Metal and Water, have all reduced.

Subjective differences between Reiki and Five Element Treatments

Here are this person's comments about how she felt the Five Element treatments differed from the many Reiki treatments that she had experienced in the past:

"In standard Reiki treatments the heat seems to build up whereas with Five Element Reiki it cools after a hot start. Energy travels round a lot (meridians?) and doesn't limit itself to area w here heat/hand is. It feels as if you are treating the problem at source, getting to grips with it, more than in a standard Reiki treatment.

"After the treatments you feel as if you've had an energy transfusion. After an emotional release the effects of Five Element Reiki tend to be more subtle and delayed, and you seem to feel flattened and unsettled for a while.

"Quite different was the sensation of being a clear glass vessel, with everything inside running smoothly and in harmony - to the extent that (this is going to sound as if I have lost it!) I was not aware of being confined in my physical body, but able to look and project outwards because it was existing effortlessly. This happened after nearly all sessions.

"Standard Reiki treatments gave a boost to my creativity but Five Element Reiki was more focused and purposeful. There was a feeling that there were no physical limits to what could be achieved.

"Like my Reiki attunements, Five Element Reiki gave me an altered perspective, a feeling of being very much part of a bigger picture."

Five Element Treatments: FAQ

I looked at my client's elements at the end of the first treatment and they are fine. Do I need to carry on with more treatments?

Yes you do. You would expect, or hope, that someone's elements will be in a balanced state by the end of a treatment, but that does not mean they will stay that way long-term.

The state of someone's elements when you first see them as a client (like the state of their chakras) reflect a trend within that person, and I don't have the impression that they flap frantically from excess to depletion from one minute to the next... unless something quite drastic like an attunement or a five element treatment happened.

When you start treating people using the five element system you will be looking at the state of their elements at weekly intervals; what happens to the elements from one day to another, from one minute to another, or from the start to the end of a treatment, is not so important.

The 'ripples' that you produce in the short term are not so important: what is important is how the elements change over a longer period, and the state that they hold after the treatments have finished.

You will need to carry out a series of treatments to produce a long term beneficial change in terms of someone's elements.

"I have been practising Five Element Reiki on a number of my regular clients and they all notice a marked difference to a regular Reiki treatment. They find it much more intense/powerful. From my point of view I find I can get down to much deeper issues."

Jeannie, England

More Advanced Treatments

Narrowing your Focus

Now we are going to make our treatment more focused.

The treatments are already focused, of course, and we have this wonderful contradiction where by narrowing our focus to deal with only one element, we are making the healing effect more intense, yet the thing that we are focusing on 'narrowly' has many associations and ramifications... so you are focusing narrowly and intensely on many things a/t the same time.

Quite a trick!

We now can go further. When you are treating the Kidney and the Bladder, say, perhaps one organ is in greater need of attention. But which organ needs more attention? You do not know at this stage.

You may have noticed a 'composite' imbalance in Water, you see, where the imbalance that you have detected is caused mainly by an imbalance in only one of the two organs.

We should remind ourselves that in reality the 'organ' is actually an energy field that exists on many levels, not just the physical organ that we immediately think of.

The "Organ Focus"

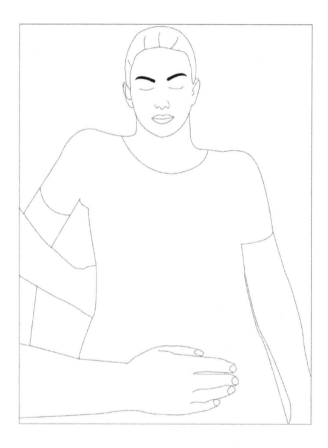

Let's imagine that you are treating Water, so your hands will be resting on the Bladder and the Kidney. While you are resting your hands in these positions you are going to use your intuition.

You are going to intuit which organ is in greater need, or to discover that both organs are in equal need. Like all things to do with intuition, there is no one set way of doing this and you may well find an approach that is different from what I am describing here.

Using imagined text

We're going to look at the state of Water in the Bladder and Kidneys. Try looking at the words Bladder and Kidneys in your mind's eye.

You might notice that one word stands out as **larger**, or in **bold type**, or in a *different font* or in a **different colour**.

One word might be smaller than the rest.

This is the organ that needs your attention. What does the other word look like? If they look the same, assume that neither has a greater need than the other.

Using a couple of sliders

It is time to bring out a small mixing desk. This time it has only two sliders. Zero is at the bottom, 100% ATTENTION! Is at the top.

One slider is for one organ, the other slider is for the other organ, say Kidney to the left and Bladder to the right.

What is your question? You are asking whether one organ or the other needs more of your attention.

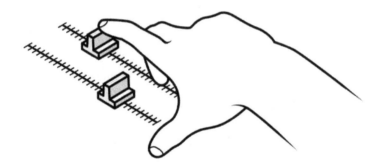

Look at the slider for Kidney; does it move? No.

Look at the slider for Bladder; does it move? Yes. It goes right up to the top.

The Bladder is in more need of attention. You need some Organ Focus...

What to do in practice

With your hands resting still on the Kidney and Bladder, in your mind's eye – with your intention – push the energy more towards the Bladder.

Focus your attention more on the Bladder than the Kidney.

You are keeping your hands on both organs because this produces the synergistic effect that we spoke about, which comes from the Japanese 'teate' system described by Michio Kushi in his book 'Macrobiotic Palm Healing'.

But you are 'leaning' more on the Bladder. Your attention is there. Your focus is there, you are dwelling more on there, and we know that the energy follows our thoughts, it follows our focus.

So in practice, when you are treating an unbalanced Water, when you feel ready you can 'look' to see whether you need to focus more on one organ than the other.

Use the Organ Focus for whatever period feels appropriate.

Other intuitive approaches

You may find that neither of these constructed images seem to feel right. In that case, use whatever intuitive approach works for you.

Maybe you don't need to imagine anything: just allow your intuition to bubble up to the surface in whatever way works best, so that you know which organ (if any) requires more attention.

A couple of ideas I could suggest would be to use an imaginary pendulum or a see-saw (teeter-totter rocker).

The imaginary pendulum could move to one side or the other to indicate the organ that needs to be focused on, or a see-saw could tilt to one side or another to indicate the same thing. If the pendulum does not move, or if the see-saw stays in a balanced state, neither organ needs extra attention.

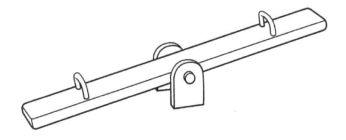

Two New Organs

Now you can deal directly with two 'Organs' that you could only allude to earlier: the Heart Protector and the Triple Heater. Earlier we always had these organs in mind when we dealt with Fire, but it was rather difficult to rest our hands on them because they are 'organs' that have no Western physical counterpart!

But we can now be more specific; we can look at them for the first time, and see if they – or one of them – need our attention.

So in practice you would glance at Heart & Small Intestine to see if one of those needed extra attention. If one of those organs needed extra attention then you would dwell on that one for a while.

When you are ready, then you can glance at the Heart Protector and Triple Heater to see if one of those needs extra attention, and react accordingly.

"Balanced Presentations"

You will not always need to focus more on one organ than another.

Sometimes you will look at the sliders and both the Yin and Yang organ will be calling for your attention equally. In that case you can carry on with the treatment approach that you learned earlier: flush energy into the organs equally from the symbol above you.

The "Aspect Focus"

We can go even deeper.

We know that by narrowing our focus we make the treatment more intense, the healing effect more profound.

By focusing on one element we have narrowed our focus and intensified the healing effect. By connecting to the organ pair we have produced a synergistic effect. By leaning on one organ we are going deeper still, but there is more…

What aspect of the organ is in greatest need of attention? Is it the physical organ? Maybe it is the emotional aspect. Maybe it's the mental state; maybe it's the spiritual aspect.

We can actually 'reach down' and 'hold' or 'cradle' the aspect of the organ that is most in need of attention.

Using a slider or scale

Imagine a scale, with a pointer that runs smoothly from the bottom to the top. Marked along the side of the scale are some legends:

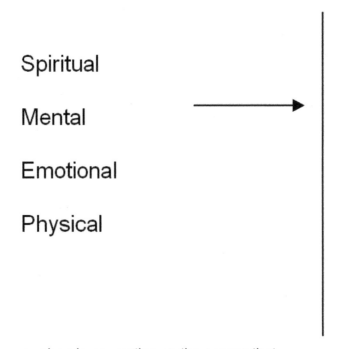

Spiritual

Mental

Emotional

Physical

So, your hands are resting on the organs that correspond to a particular element, and you have decided whether a particular 'organ' requires more attention that another.

Let's say that you are working on Metal and you notice that the Lungs are in greater need than the Large Intestine.

You focus your attention on the Lungs and in your mind's eye you look to see where the arrow settles on the sliding scale.

Maybe neither organ is in need of particular attention. That's fine: just discover which aspect of Metal should be dwelt on more.

Here is another suggestion for intuiting what aspect you need to dwell on…

Using imagined text

Try looking at the words Physical, Emotional, Mental and Spiritual in your mind's eye. You might notice that one word stands out as larger, or in bold type, or in a different font that attracts your attention.

This is the aspect that needs your attention.

Other intuitive approaches

Again, you may find that none of these constructed images seem to feel right. In that case, use whatever intuitive approach works for you. Maybe you don't need to imagine anything: just allow your intuition to bubble up to the surface in whatever way works best, so that you know which aspect of an organ (if any) requires more attention.

Which aspect of the organ in greatest need of attention? Is the mental state of the Gall Bladder the priority here? Is it the emotion of the Lungs? Is it the spiritual aspect of the Heart? Is it the physical Spleen? Maybe it's the emotion of Water or the spiritual aspect of Wood (when neither organ requires special attention).

Reach down and 'hold' or 'cradle' this aspect with your attention, with your focus. Dwell on that aspect for a while and the energy will flow with your thoughts. Stay with that until you feel that it's appropriate to move on.

Sensing the aspect

You actually may be able to sense the 'quality' of the energy that is flowing into the organ. Does the energy give the impression that it is working at the physical level, or is it working at the level of thoughts and emotions?

You can notice the nature of the energy and then dwell on that.

A Worked Example

Here is an example of someone whose elements I 'looked at' remotely the other day. I describe what I found when I looked at their elements, and talk you through a 'worked example' of what you would have done in practice if this was the person that you were treating.

This table displays the aspects that I found needed attention:

	Hollow Organ	Aspect	Solid Organ	Aspect	Bal?
Wood			**Liver**	Mental /Emotio nal*	
Fire (HT/SI)					**YES**
Fire(H P/TH)					**YES**
Earth					**YES**
Metal			**Lung**	Emotio nal	
Water	**Bladder**	Mental			

Wood

When looking at Wood, the Liver called for attention, and when I looked at the aspect the arrow hovered between thoughts and emotions, so the aspects needing attention were both the emotion of Liver (anger) and the mental state of Liver (planning). Perhaps the person is seething, suppressing their anger, or maybe they are irritable all the time, angry with themselves and other people, and they are 'stuck', unable to think coherently about the future, unable to plan.

When you treated you would rest your hands on the Liver and Gall Bladder, connect to the Wood symbol, and flush the energy through.

After a while you would look to see if an organ needed special attention, and you'd focus your attention more on the Liver.

When you felt ready, you'd reach down to and 'hold' or 'cradle' the specific aspect of the Liver that is the priority for that person on that occasion. You would have in mind the mental and emotional aspects as you merge with the Wood energy, with a beatific stillness that comes through being a clear, purposeful and focused channel.

Fire

When I looked at Fire, both physical organs called for attention, and both intangible organs called for attention, so that element would be treated in the standard way.

You would rest your hands on the Heart and Small Intestine, you would have in mind the Heart Protector and the Triple Heater, and you would let the energy flow from the Fire symbol above you.

Earth

When we looked at Earth we found that both organs were calling for our attention equally, so the treatment would again be 'standard'.

Metal

Now we move on to Metal. Here the Lungs called for attention, and the aspect that showed itself was the emotion of the Lungs, the emotion of Metal: Grief. So in practice you would be resting your hands on the Lungs and the Large Intestine, and flooding the organs with energy from the Metal symbol above you.

You would swap hands during the treatment of that element to that you connected with both left and right sides of the lungs and the large intestine.

When you felt ready you would notice that the Lungs needed more of your attention, so you would dwell on the Lungs for a while, while still connecting your hands to both 'organs'.

Then when you felt ready you would notice that it was the emotional aspect of the Lungs that were the priority here (grief) and you would 'reach down' to and 'hold' or 'cradle' that aspect, focusing your attention there, dwelling on that aspect, and as you merge with the energy it will follow your focus and be directed by your attention.

Water

Finally we move onto Water. Here the Bladder called for attention, and the mental aspect was what needed to be dwelt upon. So in practice you would be resting your hands on the Bladder and the Kidney(s), drawing energy down from the Water symbol above you.

When you felt ready you would notice that it was the Bladder that required more of your attention, so you would focus your attention more on that 'organ' and 'lean' the energy in that direction for a while.

Then when you felt comfortable you would notice that it was the mental aspect of the Bladder that was the priority, so maybe the person is mentally inflexible, or fears change in some way.

You would dwell on the mental aspect of the Bladder for whatever period felt comfortable, merging with the Water energy and letting it follow your focus.

Some Treatment Reports from Students

Report #1

"The organs needing attention were as follows:

The Liver: Mental/Emotional
The Heart and Heart Protector: Spiritual
The Spleen: Mental
The Lungs: Emotional & Spiritual

I focused on these aspects and could feel a beautiful balance taking place within the client. At this stage of working I'm not too sure if I'm doing things the way you would like me to, but I can only work with what "impressions" I receive, and I know that the more I work in this intuitive way with the 5 elemental healing technique, the stronger it will become with more clarity.

At the end of the session, the anger had dissipated and she was no longer raging about her dear husband. She did comment that this healing session felt much sharper and focused, especially around the middle of her body.

The depletion in Metal appeared to confirm her long grief with her departed sister."

Report #2

"Client came over today for treatment. She is a Reiki 1 student. Has been through a lot of heartache lately with her son.

Wood - Excess of 100%
Fire - Deficiency of 50%
Earth - Deficiency of 25%
Metal - Excess of 75%
Water - Excess of 25%

When balancing Wood, client expressed a lot of suppressed rage, which she felt ashamed of. It took a while to come into balance.

Fire element balanced fairly quickly, spreading out in wonderful gold and copper colours across the chest region.

Earth energy came in as rather coarse yet comforting and was quick to come into balance. She described it as "very heavy", as though she could not move herself.

Metal again, came down through myself as intense white/blue energy and took a wee while to balance within the client. She described it at the time as "very cold waves" moving through her.
Water balanced out in no time.

Liver: Mental/Emotional
Heart: Emotional
Spleen: Emotional
Lungs: Spiritual/Emotional
Water: Spiritual

Client released a lot of pent up resentment/anger. She is still going through a worrying time with her son who is out in Canada and has been back and forward a few times recently. "She feels helpless and powerless". She was much more composed and calmer after her healing session.

The lovely thing about this technique is, I can effortlessly merge with the energy and "become the energy. I "dance" and "move" with this beloved light as though we are one and the client then "joins" and we are all one moving wonderful force of healing colours.

There is no separation, nor are there any limitations. And this is all done with no physical movements."

Report #3

"I went along with the beautiful energies and started with the 5 element advanced technique. I am still "sparkled" by how simple and flowing this method is proving to be. I love working with these energies and sometimes I stop and say to myself, "How can it be so easy and effortless?" And back comes, "Because you have surrendered completely to the energy, therefore you are the energy, and we are as one". Isn't that wonderful? To be connected to such a loving and deep healing force, I am indeed blessed!!!"

And now back to the client...
Wood : Excess of 100%
Fire : Deficiency of 50%
Earth : Deficiency of 25%
Metal : Excess of 100%
Water : Excess of 25%

The process of bringing them into balance again was relatively simple. It took a bit longer than usual and she released a lot of emotional anger and long term suppressed rage at her "denied childhood", especially when I was working at the liver and gall bladder. (Liver screamed out for attention). Aspect focus was Mental/Emotional and I decided to use the "many hands technique" on the liver region, which proved to be somewhat powerful.

She said she could feel something very cool, almost like a soothing sensation, spreading throughout her "pain".

When working at her heart, pent up sadness was "let go". I could "see" the inner child in the foetal position crying for love and attention. And as I was balancing with the Fire energy, her anger appeared to turn to extreme hurt and rejection. Lots of sobbing.

Heart and heart protector needed attention. Aspect focus was Spiritual/Emotional. When working with the energy on these areas, she experienced something between her eyebrows, a pressure (her words).

And then lovely stillness.

Earth balanced out rather quickly. She felt a lot of "heaviness" when I was working with this energy, as though she was weighed down, but safe. Stomach needed attention. Aspect focus was physical.

Metal also took a bit to come into balance. Again I used "many hands technique" and "hui yin" to assist the balancing process. She and myself were aware of cold, blue energy coming in. She could feel it radiating through to her back. Lungs needed attention as did large intestine. Aspect focus was Emotional. Releasing again and then the blissful peace and quietness. (this lady is still in deep grief after many years, and the grief is for herself).

Water balanced out just fine. When working with this energy, there was a feeling of balance and flowing. Just completely natural. Fear will be healed and the soothing love of this universe will "always" be with us. (my impressions) bladder needed attention and the focus was again Emotional.

Finished treatment with traditional Reiki using Harmony kotodama. Emotional Butterfly at heart centre.

She felt much calmer after healing session and will certainly be back for more treatments.

Using Organ and Aspect Focus when you Self-treat

I didn't mention the Organ Focus and Aspect Focus when I wrote about self-treatments because I didn't want to make things too complicated early on and I wanted you to get used to working with the energies and experiencing their effects in a simple fashion.

Now I think you can handle these things for self-treatments!

You have learned two methods of carrying out a self-treatment in quite an intense way: the 'hands-on' and the 'hands-off' methods. For both of these methods, you can be more precise in terms of where you focus the energy.

Here's what to do: as you are focusing the energy on each element, by resting your hands and/or focusing your attention on the corresponding 'organs', just become gently aware of any organ that needs more attention than the other and let the energy flow there.

After a while, become aware of any aspect (physical, emotional, mental, spiritual) that needs attention, and allow the energy to flow there, in whatever way works for you.

Student feedback on using Organ and Aspect Focus During Self Treatments

"Just finished a self-treatment. I find the whole process very flowing, very liquid, so easy and uncluttered, like looking within myself and "seeing" what requires to be balanced and aligned!

And since working with the advanced self-healing method my dreams have given me even more insight into what needs to be addressed for further spiritual growth within myself.

Wood - In Balance
Fire - Excess of 25%
Earth - Deficiency of 25%
Metal - Excess of 100%
Water - Deficiency of 25%

When balancing Fire, strong colours of purples and blues came in, spreading throughout my whole system.

Earth felt like a gentle, yet heavy sensation bringing safety and connection to the Goddess within me.

Metal took the longest to come into balance (again). I felt an intense cold white energy tingling at my crown centre, flowing down to both lungs and around the large intestine area.

While I was "watching" this energy escaping, the feeling was tangible almost, releasing a tightness within me, and then an almost indescribable sensation of "stillness", of being on course with the whole universe. Sheer Bliss!

Water felt empowering and came into balance very quickly.

I never fail to be amazed at how simple this beautiful technique is and how gentle yet powerful these elements can come into balance through our own pure intent and visualization methods.

Focus:

Liver - Physical/Mental
Heart/H.P. - Spiritual
Stomach - Emotional
Large Intestine – Emotional
(Almost like letting go of old issues and anything which does not serve my greatest good)
Kidneys - Spiritual (the natural flow of cleansing love)"

Treating by 'pushing' some sliders

This is interesting because it demonstrates that not only can constructed visual images provide you with intuitive information, in this case the state of someone's elements, but they can also be used to effect changes in the state of someone's elements.

I am talking here about the 'mixing desk' image, with a slider for each of the five elements. Each slider runs vertically along the scale from a zero 'balance' point half way along its length: scales run up to +100% and down to -100% from that centre point.

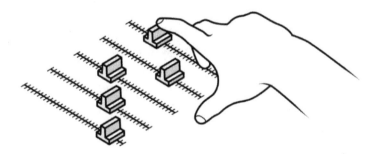

Look at the sliders in your mind's eye (or become physically aware of where the solid, heavy, metal slider are on their rails, if you aren't able to visualise too well) and notice where the excesses and deficiencies are.

With practice, you should find that you are able to do this more and more effortlessly.

Let's say there an excess of +50% in Wood.
Now, push on the slider in whatever way seems appropriate. Apply pressure, constant pressure. Notice what resistance to change the slider provides. If you need to, push harder until the slider starts to move.

Reiki will be supporting your intention, using its energy to deal with the excess and reduce it so that the slider will move down to a state of balance.

Move on to Fire. Say there's a -20% deficiency.

Push on the slider again, feel the resistance, and increase the pressure so that the slider moves up the scale. Here Reiki will boost the chi in this element to match the movement of the slider, until balance is achieved and there's nothing left to push against.

You can do this all while sitting at the head of the treatment table, with your hands resting on your client's shoulders.

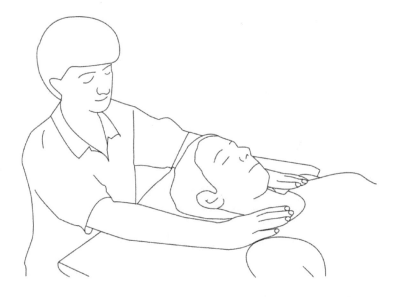

You connect to the energy and the recipient, merging with them both, you become aware of the imbalances, and guide the energy to resolve them.

Summary of Treatment Technique

The Five Element approach is based on three phases:

1. Intuiting energy imbalances in the elements
2. Stabilising and preparing the elements
3. Systematically sending each of the five energies into the associated organs

Intuiting Imbalances

There are a whole range of ways in which you can detect elemental imbalances.

You can use a prop like a pendulum or an imaginary 'slider' held in your hand, you can use constructed visual images like a virtual pendulum or a slider or a mixing desk. You could imagine text. You can allow your intuition to provide you with the necessary information in whatever way seems most easy and consistent.

You might have some insights into your client's imbalances based on what they have told you: what you know of the person, or what you can glean from what they say about their thoughts, emotions, physical problems etc.

This may help to make some sense of the imbalance you perceived, based on what you know of the various correspondences of each element.

Stabilising the Elements

Having determined which elements are most out of balance, you now need to stir things up and prepare the elements, empowering them so they can support and restrain each other in the most powerful way.

You can use a simple symbol, drawn along the length of the client's body from crown to base of spine, to open up and free up the elements. You can draw the symbol using bunched fingers or simply in your mind's eye.

Working on Organ Pairs

Now you can carry out the main part of the treatment, starting with a few minutes resting your hands on the shoulders to get Reiki flowing and bringing the client into a nice relaxed state.

If you had been detecting imbalances while sitting at the head of the treatment table with your hands on their shoulders then they are already nice and relaxed.

What you are going to do now is to connect with the pairs of 'organs' that represent each element, by resting your hands on them, and send the corresponding five element energy through them.

You will concentrate (spend more time) on the elements that were most out of balance, or the elements that you feel need more attention based on what has happened during previous treatments (the 'movements' I spoke about earlier).

You can keep track of the state of the elements intuitively as you treat, so you know when to move on.

Your treatment can be based on allowing the elemental energy to do what it needs to do to achieve balance, or you might choose to actively boost the chi in an element, or drain chi from an element, using visualisation.

Perhaps finish the treatment by resting your hands on the feet/ankles for a while, which is a nice way to bring things to a close.

And because intuition and intent/visualisation is such a powerful combination, you can even do the whole treatment in your head, without moving your hands from the shoulders!

Appendix

Recommended Reading

Traditional Acupuncture: The Law of the Five Elements
Dianne M Connelly

Macrobiotic Palm Healing
Michio Kushi with Olivia Oredson

Anyone Can Dowse for Better Health
Arthur Bailey

Web sites:

http://pipwaller.co.uk/?page_id=1281
https://www.tcmworld.org/what-is-tcm/five-elements/
https://www.pacificcollege.edu/news/blog/2016/06/22/fiv
e-elements-twelve-officials-and-causative-factor
http://www.acupuncturetoday.com/abc/fiveelementtheor
y.php

Dowsing Grid

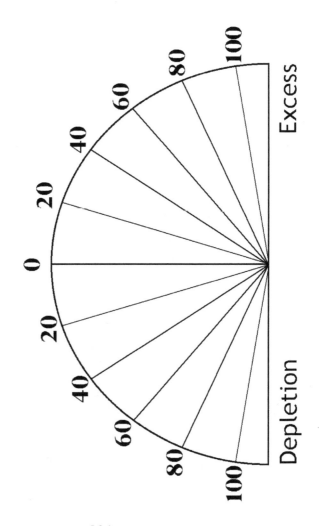